The Knowledgeable Patient

Communication and Participation in Health
A Cochrane Handbook

Contents

List of Contributors

Josip Car, Director, eHealth Unit, Department of Primary Care and Public Health, Faculty of Medicine, Imperial College London, London, United Kingdom

Helen Dilkes, Research Officer, Health Knowledge Network, Centre for Health Communication and Participation, Australian Institute for Primary Care and Ageing, La Trobe University, Bundoora, Victoria, Australia

Mary Draper, Independent Healthcare Consultant, Victoria, Australia

Adrian G.K. Edwards, Professor in General Practice, Department of Primary Care and Public Health, School of Medicine, Cardiff University, Cardiff, Wales, United Kingdom

Sophie Hill, Coordinating Editor/Head, Cochrane Consumers and Communication Review Group, Centre for Health Communication and Participation, Australian Institute for Primary Care and Ageing, La Trobe University, Bundoora, Victoria, Australia

Dell Horey, Research Fellow, Division of Health Research, Faculty of Health Sciences, La Trobe University, Bundoora, Victoria, Australia

Maureen Johnson, Manager, Women's Consumer Health Information, The Royal Women's Hospital, Parkville, Victoria, Australia

Jessica Kaufman, Research Officer, Cochrane Consumers and Communication Review Group, Centre for Health Communication and Participation, Australian Institute for Primary Care and Ageing, La Trobe University, Bundoora, Victoria, Australia

John Kis-Rigo, Trials Search Coordinator, Cochrane Consumers and Communication Review Group, Centre for Health Communication and Participation, Australian Institute for Primary Care and Ageing, La Trobe University, Bundoora, Victoria, Australia

Simon Lewin, Senior Researcher, Preventive and International Health Care Unit, Norwegian Knowledge Centre for the Health Services, Oslo,

Norway; Health Systems Research Unit, Medical Research Council of South Africa, Cape Town, South Africa

Chaojie Liu, School of Public Health, La Trobe University, Bundoora, Victoria, Australia

Dianne B. Lowe, Research Officer, Cochrane Consumers and Communication Review Group, Centre for Health Communication and Participation, Australian Institute for Primary Care and Ageing, La Trobe University, Bundoora, Victoria, Australia

Joanne E. McKenzie, School of Public Health and Preventive Medicine, Monash University, Melbourne, Victoria, Australia

Brian McKinstry, Professor of Primary Care E-Health, Centre for Population Health Sciences, University of Edinburgh, Edinburgh, Scotland, United Kingdom

Sandy Oliver, Professor of Public Policy, Social Science Research Unit and EPPI-Centre, Institute of Education, University of London, London, United Kingdom

Yannis Pappas, Deputy Director, eHealth Unit, Department of Primary Care and Public Health, Faculty of Medicine, Imperial College London, London, United Kingdom

Megan Prictor, Managing Editor, Cochrane Consumers and Communication Review Group, Centre for Health Communication and Participation, Australian Institute for Primary Care and Ageing, La Trobe University, Bundoora, Victoria, Australia

Rebecca E. Ryan, Research Fellow, Cochrane Consumers and Communication Review Group, Centre for Health Communication and Participation, Australian Institute for Primary Care and Ageing, La Trobe University, Bundoora, Victoria, Australia

Nancy Santesso, Department of Clinical Epidemiology and Biostatistics, McMaster University, Hamilton, Canada

Ruth Stewart, ESRC Research Fellow, Social Science Research Unit, Institute of Education, University of London, London, United Kingdom

Preface

A Google search of 'knowledgeable patient' brings up all the change and flux of the last century. If I take the words of the google search result at face value, what are my thoughts?[1]

> 'Investigating the role of lay knowledge' *(leading me to wonder, does the patient know something that the doctor does not?)*
>
> 'A beautiful woman goes to the gynaecologist' *(patients (and women) are still the butt of jokes)*
>
> 'Your first knowledgeable patient' *(doctors confront people with knowledge – and questions!)*
>
> 'Compliant . . . the patient needs to be educated – by us – to understand why he needs to follow our instructions' *(the patient knows nothing and must be obedient)*
>
> 'Inside the mind of . . .' *(we have to take knowledgeable patients seriously)*

In the twentieth century, patients moved from passivity to participation, and like all major social change, movement was uneven. Being more involved may also mean being more responsible for one's health. This is a public policy dilemma because being sick can lead to vulnerability,

---

[1] www.google.com.au. I searched with 'knowledgeable patient' on 26 June 2009. The extracts are taken from the first five listings of the search result, with the source material being:

'Investigating. . .' Karlsson M (2007) *The knowledgeable patient: investigating the role of lay knowledge in the production of health.* www.ageing.ox.ac.uk/files/workingpaper_208.pdf.

'A beautiful. . .' hnbaby (2007) *Medical Geek Forum.* www.medicalgeek.com/medicaljokes/7025-knowledgeable-patient.html.

'Your. . .' Blades K (2004) *Pulse.* www.pulsetoday.co.uk/article-content/-/article_display_list/10899114/your-first-knowledgeable-patient.

'Compliant. . .' Romano PE (1987) *Archives of Ophthalmology.* http://archopht.ama-assn.org/cgi/reprint/105/3/315-a.pdf.

'Inside. . .' Dillon B (2008) *Geovoices: Geonetric Blog.* http://geovoices.wordpress.com/2008/05/06/inside-the-mind-of-the-cancer-patient.

and speaking up may not be the priority for the sick person. It confronts us with the test of fairness because poorer people have more ill health than those who are well off materially and socially.

In the twenty-first century, the pressures of this change are apparent. 'Ordinary' people have to be extraordinary. Much is expected: keep up to date with screening, know your medicines, recognise the latest risks, manage the family's health, eat sensibly, exercise, plan for end of life, understand your insurance options and communicate your wishes. And possibly contribute to your community by volunteering your time and support.

The 'knowledgeable patient', then, is sometimes a patient, sometimes a family carer, sometimes a member of the public interested in health issues, sometimes a consumer advocate, contributing to the health system or to a healthier society – and sometimes all of these things. In other words, the knowledgeable patient is fundamental to improving health and managing illness.

Being more knowledgeable creates a new dynamic in the health system. The knowledgeable patient may create demand, ask questions and seek information. Expectations on people may be too high, though, and people could get lost in confusion, preyed on by unscrupulous parties promoting the latest cure-all. Simply, the health system may be too busy to answer questions, or not able to comprehend the complex demands it faces.

This book sits at the forefront of these changes. It will be an essential guide for the new era of complex healthcare. Its purpose is to help health professionals to understand the vital relationship they will have with the 'knowledgeable patient' and equip them to contribute to a new form of health system, based on evidence of effective and responsive strategies for improving communication and participation.

The book is for people who are interested in a 'consumer-perspective' on health issues. Those who are training to be health professionals or coming back to study for postgraduate education are an important audience. It is relevant to a broad group, such as those training for clinical roles in health or medicine, or those undertaking education in public health, health policy, health administration or health information management. Another important audience are those who want to read patient stories and who want to know the evidence behind strategies to communicate better and involve people in health.

The book contains a wealth of issues for exploration and discussion, with many different health examples – safe medicine use, chronic disease self-management, surgery, the complexity of multimorbidity and rare disease risk. It contributes research to our growing understanding of knowledge transfer, i.e. getting research into health practice and into people's lives. New issues in health – public involvement in research, emerging health communication technologies and health literacy – are documented. Research examples are not confined to one service domain but span living in the community, health service treatment, governance and policy making.

It is international in scope, giving readers ideas, concepts, taxonomies, evidence and practical tools to understand the central role of communication and participation to a well-functioning health system. It draws on several research paradigms, presenting qualitative research of experiences for integrating with evidence from systematic reviews of controlled trials.

It places communication and participation firmly in the future of evidence-based healthcare. It gives us a language to communicate a better future.

Sophie Hill, Editor
Australian Institute for Primary Care and Ageing, La Trobe University,
Bundoora, Victoria, Australia
June 2011

Acknowledgements

This book was made possible by a grant from the Policy and Strategy Unit, Quality, Safety and Patient Experience Branch, Department of Health, Victoria, Australia. In particular, I acknowledge the vision and support of Ms Alison McMillan and Ms Catherine Harmer, senior officers with the Department. The grant supported involvement in the book by staff in the Centre for Health Communication and Participation (CHCP), at the Australian Institute for Primary Care and Ageing, La Trobe University. Additionally, the work of the Cochrane Consumers and Communication Review Group (CC&CRG), which is situated in CHCP, has been supported by the Department of Health Victoria through a Health Service and Funding Agreement since 2000. Many of the ideas and concepts developed in the book have grown from the editorial work of the Group, particularly for Chapters 1–4 and 8–12. The Victorian Department of Health has therefore made a major contribution to building the evidence base for better communication with and involvement by consumers in health.

I also acknowledge the Australian Department of Health and Ageing for successive grants to the CC&CRG since 2001 for Infrastructure funding, Funding for Australian-based Cochrane Collaboration Activities, which have supported work discussed in Chapters 7, 9 and 10.

I give thanks to many collaborators for the concepts and research presented in Chapters 3 and 4. In Chapter 3, the concept of the multidirectional nature of health communication grew out of collaboration with Professor Sandy Oliver, EPPI Centre, University of London, who is a member of the editorial team for the CC&CRG. In earlier work, when we were articulating the scope of interventions covered by the Review Group and organising them more logically into groups, Sandy emphasised the importance of communication *from* consumers and the need for health professionals to listen to patients and health consumers in a more formal sense. Ms Judy Stoelwinder, the then Trials Search Coordinator of the CC&CRG, developed the coding scheme used to quantify the trials and direction of communication and participation in Table 3.1. Judy also made a substantial contribution to the development of the taxonomy of outcomes discussed in Chapter 4 and her pioneering work in this field is most gratefully acknowledged. Dr Adrian Edwards, Professor in General Practice at Cardiff University, read Chapter 3 to ensure that the description of risk communication interventions made clinical sense. The research to develop the medicines interventions taxonomy described in Table 3.2 was made possible through two grants from the Canadian Agency for Drugs and Technologies in Health, 2006–2010, PI Professor

J Grimshaw, in the Rx for Change database project. Table 3.2 is adapted from Lowe D, Ryan R, Santesso N, Hill S. (2010) Development of a taxonomy of interventions to organise the evidence on consumers' medicines use, *Patient Education and Counseling* DOI: 10.1016/j.pec.2010.09.024, with permission of Elsevier, Copyright © 2010, Elsevier Publishing. In Chapter 3, I define interventions for communication and participation as purposeful, planned and formalised strategies associated with a diverse range of intentions or aims. The provenance for this concept is that I first presented it at a Plenary (A.E.I.O.U. of Communication and Participation', Hill S, Prictor M. 4th Australasian Conference on Quality and Safety, Melbourne, 21–23 August 2006). A condensed outline was published in *Communicating with consumers and carers – Part 1 – Pilot of evidence-based selection of communication strategies to improve communication between consumers/carers and health services,* Victorian Quality Council, 2007; and which is reproduced with permission (refer to Chapter 15 below). Chapter 3 extends the concept and combines it with the concept of multi-directionality, which was first published in 2009, Hill S, Directions in health communication, *Bulletin of the World Health Organization,* 87, 648.

The research conducted in Chapter 5 was part of a larger study funded by the Australian Department of Health and Ageing and conducted for the National Vascular Disease Prevention Alliance, 2003–2004. I acknowledge Professor Andrew Tonkin, Monash University, Australia, who conceived and designed the original study.

The fieldwork for the doctoral thesis which formed part of Chapter 6 was supported by a research grant from the Victorian Health Promotion Foundation, Project no 96-0858, 1997–1999, PI Dr J. Daly.

Chapter 7 drew from research supported by a Public Health Research grant, Department of Human Services Victoria, 2006–2007, PI Dr C Mead.

I acknowledge La Trobe University Faculty of Health Sciences Grant (2007) for support underpinning Chapter 14. In addition, Rebecca Ryan and I acknowledge our colleagues Dr Klara Brunnhuber, BMJ Evidence Centre, London, and Dr James Woodcock, London School of Hygiene and Tropical Medicine, for the collaboration on multimorbidity, extending our ideas further.

Where derived from the original reports, the material in Chapter 15 is Copyright © State of Victoria, Australia and reproduced with permission of the Victorian Minister for Health. Unauthorised reproduction and other uses comprised in the copyright are prohibited without permission. The knowledge translation research in Chapter 15 was funded by the Victorian Quality Council in 2004, and conducted with a major commitment from the staff at the Royal Women's Hospital. The Project Officer at the CC&CRG was Ms Angela Melder and her contribution to the project's successful conduct is gratefully acknowledged.

The concepts around health literacy presented in Chapter 16 were first developed in two papers. I would like to thank the following for the opportunity to explore the issues: the Australian Department of Health and Ageing and the Cochrane Collaboration Policy Liaison Network for a forum in Canberra on health literacy in 2008; and the National Medicines Policy Partnership for their Forum in Sydney June 2010.

The activities and resources described in Chapter 17 were supported by two sources: a grant to the CC&CRG under the Evaluating the Effectiveness of Participation scheme, Department of Human Services of Victoria, Australia, 2007–2008; and a grant from the Helen McPherson Smith Trust in 2007–08 for the establishment of the Health Knowledge Network.

In Chapter 18, Table 18.2 is adapted with permission from Professor Aziz Sheikh, and first published in Catwell L, Sheikh A. (2009) Evaluating eHealth interventions: the need for continuous systemic evaluation. *Public Library of Science Medicine*. **6**, e1000126.

The book has several figures that capture concepts and ideas so well, it makes the words redundant! So I would like to acknowledge and thank Helen Dilkes for her original work for Figures 2.1, 2.2, 16.1 and 17.1–17.3. I thank and acknowledge Jessica Kaufman for Figure 7.1 and Dianne Lowe for Figures 9.1 and 9.2.

A few special people helped make the book a reality. Jessica Kaufman and Dianne Lowe, authors of many of the chapters, generously provided many extra hours of assistance in the background. It has been a pleasure to work with such wonderful young researchers. Jessica Thomas came to work with us for four months in 2010 as Managing Editor of the CC&CRG and she helped enormously with editing and organisation. And my brother Tom Hill helped me find the words to write the 'first page'.

Finally, my thanks go to Wiley-Blackwell, in particular Mary Banks, Senior Publisher, and Jon Peacock, Development Editor, who remained so encouraging and supportive along the way.

Sophie Hill, Editor

CHAPTER 1
Does communication with consumers and carers need to improve?

Megan Prictor[1] *and Sophie Hill*[2]
[1]Managing Editor, Cochrane Consumers and Communication Review Group, Centre for Health Communication and Participation, Australian Institute for Primary Care and Ageing, La Trobe University, Bundoora, Victoria, Australia
[2]Coordinating Editor/Head, Cochrane Consumers and Communication Review Group, Centre for Health Communication and Participation, Australian Institute for Primary Care and Ageing, La Trobe University, Bundoora, Victoria, Australia

The stories we solicited reverberated with recurring and troubling themes: You cannot get a human being on the telephone, and you cannot get an appointment. When you do have an appointment, you wait an excessive time before seeing the doctor, who is in a hurry, does not seem to care, and provides inadequate explanation and education .... Each event had the potential to weaken the patient's relationship with the clinician and culminate in loss of trust in the health care system [1].

When my (MP) daughter was aged about 3, after a series of colds she was referred to a specialist for advice on mild fluid on the ears. This experience, although she does not remember it, shook my confidence in the health system. Things got off to a poor start when the specialist, who happened to be male and probably in his fifties, did not greet my daughter nor ask my name (preferring to call me 'mum'), and did not introduce himself until prompted. Without a hearing test, after a brief look in her ears, he pronounced that she needed surgery to insert grommets to drain the fluid; that I would be grateful and would thank him once it was done; and that he could squeeze us in 2 days before Christmas. Rather taken aback, I enquired about possible risks or side effects of the procedure and was informed there were none. When I suggested I would rather take a 'wait-and-see' approach, he warned me not to stick my

The Knowledgeable Patient: Communication and Participation in Health – A Cochrane Handbook, First Edition. Edited by Sophie Hill.

head in the sand and that adverse consequences would likely follow. After the appointment, I sought a second opinion and did not proceed with surgery.

I am an educated white female in my thirties, working for an organisation that conducts research into what makes for good doctor–patient communication. I had read about the health problem and the procedure beforehand, so had a good idea that what the specialist was telling me was not quite correct. Although there were no practical adverse consequences (i.e. my daughter was not subjected to unnecessary surgery), the experience left me so shaken that afterwards I burst into tears, and years later, it stayed with me. And I wondered about the parents of other patients of this specialist – did some of them also harbour doubts, but accepted his recommendations because he similarly implied that they were bad parents if they failed to heed his advice? Did they accept being treated rudely because, after all, he was the doctor?

What is the broader health policy and social context?

It could be argued that treatment effectiveness – whether a particular medicine or surgery works to improve life of the patient – is more important than whether the patient feels good about their relationship with their doctor, whether they are well informed about their treatment and whether they have been involved in decision-making. This might be particularly claimed in resource-poor or crisis settings, where efforts must focus unambiguously on the preservation of life [2]. In the bigger picture, my experience of poor communication with the specialist is arguably of very little consequence.

It is now well established, however, that good communication is fundamental to healthcare, both of itself and as a mechanism to ensure safe, effective treatment. This chapter establishes the case for efforts to improve communication between healthcare professionals and patients. It identifies how we can find out about the nature and extent of communication problems, and most importantly, what the consequences of these problems are. By demonstrating that communication-related difficulties affect not only people's feelings but also the quality, efficacy and safety of the medical and surgical treatments they receive, we establish that attempts to overcome the difficulties are more than just feel-good strategies. Rather, they are critical to improving people's health and ensuring that medical mistakes are avoided.

How do we find out about communication problems?

Data on communication difficulties in healthcare settings are available in diverse locations. Discussions of healthcare quality and safety often circle around these issues. Observational data are routinely collected by hospitals and healthcare quality agencies. For instance in Victoria, Australia, public hospital data on adult inpatients are gathered annually using the Victorian Patient Satisfaction Monitor, a tool which incorporates measures of (1) written and oral provision of information to patients about the hospital, treatment, medications and at discharge; (2) staff attitudes, responsiveness and communication; and (3) complaints management [3]. Stories about the impact of communication problems on patients, their families and clinicians also make it into the mainstream literature. Nancy Berlinger's paper on people's experiences of communication around medical error draws on narratives published in books, journals, general magazines and the internet [4]. Indeed, the focus on medical mistakes and adverse events heralded by the landmark 2000 Institute of Medicine report *To Err Is Human: Building a Safer Health System* arguably lends weight to research and discussion of patient involvement and improved clinician–patient interaction, since there is growing evidence – discussed below – that they are more than merely window dressing.

Healthcare complaints data, which are sometimes publicly reported, are the key to better understanding these issues. Poor communication itself is a major stimulus for complaints to hospitals and monitoring bodies. People may feel that they have been treated discourteously or given insufficient or incorrect information [5]. The US Agency for Healthcare Research and Quality noted that in 2005, for instance, almost one in ten adults reported poor communication when using health services in the previous year [6]. Significantly, poor communication was reported more often by people from racial and ethnic minority groups and those on lower incomes [7]. A study of people who had made complaints to hospitals in the Netherlands had similar findings, whereby 9% of these complaints were solely about communication between doctors and patients [8]. Obviously, diverse coding taxonomies result in different findings; however, there is no reason to expect the picture is any better in Australia. A study of 1308 complaints made at a major South Australian hospital over a 30-month period found that fully 45% ($n = 621$) of complaints were about communication problems, comprising a lack of communication ($n = 240$), offensive attitude ($n = 124$), lack of care ($n = 112$), inadequate information ($n = 98$), conflicting information ($n = 47$) and undignified service ($n = 6$) [9, 10].

Complaints data also reveal that communication failures underpin many other types of health system problems. The Victorian Health Services Commissioner noted in 2008 that 'communication is a feature of all complaints' – whether they fall into the 'communication' category or not [5], whilst in West Australia, many of the complaints categorised as relating to treatment or access also related to the provision of information and effective consultation [11]. In the Dutch study, most complaints (68%) were about the clinical conduct of healthcare professionals 'frequently in combination with shortcomings in relational conduct or shortcomings in the information provided by the professional' [8].

Communication problems matter to patients

In the example above, poor communication had no impact other than that I felt upset and angry. I did not see it as part of a broader problem. Yet poor communication in the healthcare setting is very common. Personal accounts give some indication that poor communication can have a severe and lasting impact on people's experiences. In a recent paper about rare diseases, the mother of a child with fragile X syndrome described as 'the hell of my life' not the child's illness itself, but rather the clumsy and insensitive diagnosis disclosure by the physician [12].

Kuzel and colleagues, in a 2004 paper, pointed out that the focus on medical errors – such as medication and surgical mistakes in inpatient settings – highlighted by the *To Err Is Human* report is at odds with the types of problems that patients generally describe in encountering the health system. Patients in primary care are more likely to talk about difficulties in the doctor–patient relationship (primarily disrespect or insensitivity) and access difficulties, which overwhelmingly cause them psychological or emotional harms – including anger, frustration and loss of trust – as well as physical harm (particularly pain) and financial cost [1]. This is supported by Commonwealth Fund surveys showing that access difficulties, and breakdowns in care coordination and information flow, were experienced by most US adults [13, 14].

There is clear evidence that people want more information than they are given and that clinicians tend to overestimate the amount of information they have provided [15, 16]. Roter and Makoul have noted that only 58% of people studied said their healthcare provider told them things in a way they could understand [17]. Unsurprisingly, communication difficulties have been shown to affect diagnosis: Stewart noted that '50% of psychosocial and psychiatric problems are missed, that physicians interrupted patients an average of 18 seconds into the patient's description of the presenting problem, that 54% of patient problems and 45% of patient concerns are neither elicited by the physician nor disclosed by the patient' [18].

Adverse events

Communication failures can cause not only dissatisfaction but serious adverse events (an 'injury caused by medical care' [19]). In 2008–2009, the report on such events in Victorian hospitals identified that communication was a contributing factor in 20% of these events, with health information a factor in another 8% of cases [20]. Similarly a US review of adverse events in obstetrics and gynaecology identified communication failures – either between clinicians or between clinicians and patients – as being associated with 31% of these events [21]. Communication failures between clinicians and patients contribute to wrong-site surgery, in which surgery is conducted on the wrong part of the body, the wrong surgery is done or the wrong patient is operated on [22]. Not communicating well with patients and their families and not including the patient or family in identifying the right surgical site are key causal factors in this type of error [23]. The World Health Organization's Surgical Safety Checklist for clinicians includes, as a necessary first step, that the patient has confirmed his or her identify, the surgical site and the surgical procedure, and given his or her consent [24].

A classic definition of medical error from the research literature is 'failure of a planned action to be completed as intended or the use of a wrong plan to achieve an aim' [25]. People using healthcare, however, have a broader conception of the term. Gallagher, Burroughs and colleagues have identified that patients see medical errors as including communication problems such as being treated rudely, poor responsiveness on the part of the clinician and long waiting times [25, 26]. Researchers portray this conception of medical errors as being plainly wrong, a misunderstanding on the part of patients. Consequently, the authors call for doctors to explain more clearly to patients the 'correct' meaning of the term 'medical error'. This so-called misunderstanding by patients could, instead, stimulate a broad reconceptualisation of the term to encompass the things that patients are concerned about and see as wrong in healthcare, such as access and communication difficulties. If, as Kuzel and others have identified, being treated offhandedly and not being able to see a doctor loom large in people's concerns about the health system, there must be a greater emphasis on addressing communication problems seriously and systematically. As Kuzel notes, 'respectful communication should not be an optional extra in healthcare. Studies of patients' or service users' experiences and perspectives allow us to recognize more readily that hurtful comments are harmful comments and that failures of respect can be both unhelpful and damaging to health' [27].

Litigation

Poor communication is known to be a key contributing factor in litigation against primary care physicians [28]. Moreover, in circumstances in which an adverse event has already occurred, clear communication becomes critical [29]. A recent study about open-disclosure policies in Australian hospitals found that 'how patients were treated, whether their experiences were valued and whether their questions were answered truthfully influenced patients' judgements about the merit of the process' [29]. In a US study of parents who filed malpractice claims for perinatal injuries, those who felt misled or not sufficiently well informed by the healthcare provider about their child's problems and their cause were more likely to sue even if the care provided had been technically adequate [30].

How can things be improved?

There is growing recognition of the importance of communication and participation in healthcare. There is a substantial body of research – conducted particularly by researchers in the United Kingdom, Western Europe, USA, Canada and Australia – into better ways to communicate with and involve people in their health management and healthcare delivery and planning. Health literacy interventions, self-management programmes, written information, new communication technologies, empathetic communication styles and the involvement of family care-givers are among the wide-ranging research streams that have been the focus of attention and funding.

Recognition of the significance of effective communication in the healthcare context was highlighted by the 1997 establishment of a review group within the internationally recognised Cochrane Collaboration, focusing on this topic. The Cochrane Consumers and Communication Review Group (www.latrobe.edu.au/chcp/cochrane) facilitates systematic reviews of interventions which affect consumers' interactions with healthcare professionals, services and researchers (see Box 1.1). The interventions may relate, for example, to individual use of healthcare services or to consumer participation in health planning, policy and research (discussed further in Chapter 2). This places communication – and poor communication – in a new context, that of evidence-based healthcare. All of the authors of this book are involved in the Cochrane Consumers and Communication Review Group, as editors, researchers, referees and collaborating colleagues.

The scope of the book

This book is about the importance of knowledgeable patients in all their various roles and regardless of their label – as patients, consumers, carers, lay persons, peers, volunteers or advocates – and how they contribute to the creation of a healthier society. It is about the importance of communication and participation at all levels, from individual through to collective contexts.

One of the aims of the book is to inform and educate health professionals and equip them with the resources to explore these issues further. It places communication and participation firmly into the context of evidence-based healthcare, explaining what this means and why it is relevant to practice and policy.

Box 1.1 Systematic reviews

You are browsing the newspaper and read about the results of a controlled clinical trial. The trial's conclusions are positive – the treatment 'Now Even Better' has been shown to work and is described as the best choice. Six months later, you read that a new trial has concluded that 'Now Even Better' is no more effective than 'Now Better', which has been around for many years and is cheaper. (Side effects are not described in either article.) Which piece of research do you believe? This dilemma faces health professionals and consumers all the time, and is increasingly problematic as more research is conducted.

Systematic reviews of interventions are major types of research. In a systematic review, all the findings of controlled clinical trials of a specific intervention are collated and summarised to find out if on average the intervention works [31]. The aim is to provide a conclusive summary and synthesis so that decision-makers – whether they are health professionals, consumers or policy makers – can make a decision informed by all the relevant research on the topic.

This book provides information about all facets of systematic reviews of interventions for communication and participation. All chapters reference relevant Cochrane systematic reviews (i.e. reviews prepared by people involved in The Cochrane Collaboration and published on *The Cochrane Library*, www.cochrane.org). Chapter 2 gives a summary of evidence-based healthcare and the role of systematic reviews; Chapter 3 describes what interventions are; and Chapter 4 outlines the range of outcomes from communication and participation interventions. In Chapter 8, stories from consumers on how they used Cochrane reviews for personal decisions are presented, and the chapter includes a guide to all sections of a Cochrane review. Chapter 9 aims to quantify the systematic reviews relevant to improving health systems. Chapter 12 shows how to get the most from Cochrane reviews.

The book has four sections:

1: What are the benefits of improving people's participation in their health through effective interaction?

Chapters 1–4 establish the scope of the book and provide the conceptual building blocks and practical knowledge tools.

Chapter 1 has provided the justification for why action to improve communication with consumers and measures to support their involvement are worth pursuing.

Chapter 2 advances an overarching conceptual framework, situates the book in the context of the evidence-based healthcare movement and provides key definitions and terms.

Chapter 3 defines interventions for communication and participation and includes a case study of interventions for safe medicine use.

Chapter 4 looks at the types of outcomes resulting from interventions that promote knowledgeable and involved consumers and carers. It looks at what outcomes have been measured in the past and proposes a new taxonomy of outcomes of importance to consumers of interventions for improving communication and participation.

2: What do people want from communication and participation in health?

Chapters 5–8 present research findings from qualitative research into people's experiences of health and identify what consumers and carers want in terms of communication and participation.

Chapter 5 explores the different ways in which absolute risk for cardiovascular disease can be discussed by consumers and general practitioners in primary care settings.

Chapter 6 examines consumer participation from the patient's perspective. It draws from in-depth interviews with people who had carotid endarterectomy surgery to identify three major participation patterns.

Chapter 7 outlines the findings of a systematic review of the experiences, views and needs of people at medically acquired risk for Creutzfeldt–Jakob disease (CJD) and variant CJD and presents a framework which identifies how communication might best happen in these situations.

Chapter 8 presents research with consumers about how they used evidence from systematic reviews in planning and managing their health.

3: Where is the evidence: information sources, skills and tools for health professionals and consumers?

Not only are we bombarded with information but increasingly we are confronted by new health research. The field of evidence on improving communication and participation is no different. When should we look, what will we find and how should we use research? These questions are addressed in Chapters 9–12.

Chapter 9 combines two concepts in order to identify the scope and quantity of evidence for improving health and the experience of treatment. The first concept is termed evidence for health systems decision-making and the second is evidence to promote health and improve the experience of illness and treatment.

Chapter 10 takes a critical perspective to the topic of online health literacy and looks at how users can be misled. The implications for a realistic assessment of educational strategies to achieve the 'autonomous' patient are discussed.

Chapter 11 reviews and discusses the current evidence and future research agenda for educational interventions directed to health professionals and consumers to improve their ability to communicate with one another.

Chapter 12 looks at examples of how Cochrane reviews can provide evidence that is relevant to different audiences and how it is used by them.

4: How to build capacity for a health system focused on communication and participation?

Chapters 13–18 conclude the book by drawing from research into knowledge transfer and health reform processes to provide lessons for future actions.

Chapter 13 considers how research is funded and the opportunities this presents for involving patients and the wider public in deciding what problems deserve research and how that research should be done.

Chapter 14 examines the emerging issue of multimorbidity, i.e. having more than one health problem. It examines what evidence exists to support the use of evidence-based interventions for communication and participation in the area of medicines where people have more than one health condition.

Chapter 15 contributes to the growing literature on evidence-informed health service improvement by examining how research on communication was integrated into a service improvement project at a major women's hospital in Victoria, Australia.

Chapter 16 discusses the concept of health literacy and its relation to evidence-based healthcare and draws on submissions to a major national health reform process to identify how different players and health organisations want health literacy improved.

Chapter 17 describes healthcare intervention trials, research evaluation, knowledge transfer and capacity building, and the international initiatives putting these concepts into practice.

Chapter 18 introduces the reader to an array of health information technologies that may facilitate patient communication, discusses the potential of these technologies to improve healthcare through improved communication and participation, and outlines the challenges of implementing communication technologies.

References

1. Kuzel AJ, Woolf SH, Gilchrist VJ, et al. (2004) Patient reports of preventable problems and harms in primary health care. *Annals of Family Medicine* **2**, 333–340.
2. Edwards A, Elwyn G (2001) Evidence-based patient choice. In: Edwards A, Elwyn G, (eds.) *Evidence-Based Patient Choice: Inevitable or Impossible*. Oxford University Press, Oxford, pp. 3–4.
3. Department of Health Victoria (2009) *Your Hospitals: A Report on Victoria's Public Hospitals. July 2008 to June 2009*. Department of Health Victoria, Melbourne.

4. Berlinger N (2003) Broken stories: patients, families, and clinicians after medical error. *Literature and Medicine* **22**, 230–240.
5. Office of Health Services Commissioner (2008) *2008 Annual Report*. Office of Health Services Commissioner, Victoria.
6. Agency for Healthcare Research and Quality (2008) *National Healthcare Quality Report.* US Department of Health and Human Services. Available from: http://www.ahrq.gov/qual/qrdr08.htm. Accessed: 23 February 2010.
7. Agency for Healthcare Research and Quality (2008) *National Healthcare Disparities Report 2008.* US Department of Health and Human Services. Available from: http://www.ahrq.gov/qual/qrdr08.htm. Accessed: 23 February 2010.
8. Friele RD, Sluijs EM (2006) Patient expectations of fair complaint handling in hospitals: empirical data. *BMC Health Services Research* **6**, 106.
9. Anderson K, Allan D, Finucane P (2001) A 30-month study of patient complaints at a major Australian hospital. *Journal of Quality in Clinical Practice* **21**, 109–111.
10. Wofford MM, Wofford JL, Bothra J, Kendrick SB, Smith A, Lichstein PR (2004) Patient complaints about physician behaviors: a qualitative study. *Academic Medicine* **79**, 134–138.
11. Office of Health Review WA (2009) *Annual Report 2008–09*. Office of Health Review, Perth. Available from: http://www.healthreview.wa.gov.au/publications/docs/2008-09%20Annual%20Report_68.pdf. Accessed: 23 February 2010.
12. Huyard C (2009) What, if anything, is specific about having a rare disorder? Patients' judgements on being ill and being rare. *Health Expectations* **12**, 361–370.
13. Schoen C, Osborn R, How S, Doty M, Peugh J (2008) In chronic condition: experiences of patients with complex health care needs, in eight countries. *Health Affairs Web Exclusive*. Available from: http://www.commonwealthfund.org/Content/Publications/In-the-Literature/2008/Nov/In-Chronic-Condition–Experiences-of-Patients-with-Complex-Health-Care-Needs–in-Eight-Countries–20.aspx. Accessed: February 23, 2010.
14. How S, Shih A, Lau J, Schoen C (2008) *Public Views on US Health System Organisation: A Call for New Directions*. Available from: http://www.commonwealthfund.org/Content/Publications/Data-Briefs/2008/Aug/Public-Views-on-U-S–Health-System-Organization–A-Call-for-New-Directions.aspx. Accessed: 23 February 2010.
15. Rosenberg EE, Lussier MT, Beaudoin C (1997) Lessons for clinicians from physician-patient communication literature. *Archives of Family Medicine* **6**, 279–283.
16. Kinnersley P, Edwards A, Hood K, et al. (2007) Interventions before consultations for helping patients address their information needs. *Cochrane Database of Systematic Reviews*, CD004565.
17. Roter D, Makoul G (2003) *Objective 11-6: Healthcare Providers' Communication Skills. Healthy People 2010*. US Department of Health and Human Services, Washington DC.
18. Stewart MA (1995) Effective physician-patient communication and health outcomes: a review. *Canadian Medical Association Journal* **152**, 1423–1433.
19. AHRQ. *Patient Safety Network. Glossary*. Available from: http://www.psnet.ahrq.gov/glossary.aspx. Accessed: 23 February 2010.
20. Department of Health Victoria (2009) *Building Foundations to Support Patient Safety: Annual Report of the 2008–09 Sentinel Event Program*. Department of Health, Victoria.

21. White AA, Pichert JW, Bledsoe SH, Irwin C, Entman SS (2005) Cause and effect analysis of closed claims in obstetrics and gynecology. *Obstetrics and Gynecology* **105**, 1031–1038.
22. Hughes R (ed.) (2008) *Patient Safety and Quality: An Evidence-Based Handbook for Nurses*. Agency for Healthcare Research and Quality, MD.
23. Mulloy D, Hughes R (2008) Wrong-site surgery: a preventable medical error. In: Hughes R, (ed.) *Patient Safety and Quality: An Evidence-Based Handbook for Nurses*. Agency for Healthcare Research and Quality, MD.
24. World Health Organization (2009) *WHO Surgical Safety Checklist*. Available from: http://www.who.int/patientsafety/safesurgery/tools_resources/en/index.html. Accessed: 23 February 2010.
25. Gallagher TH, Waterman AD, Ebers AG, Fraser VJ, Levinson W (2003) Patients' and physicians' attitudes regarding the disclosure of medical errors. *Journal of the American Medical Association* **289**, 1001–1007.
26. Burroughs TE, Waterman AD, Gallagher TH, et al. (2007) Patients' concerns about medical errors during hospitalization. *Joint Commission Journal on Quality and Patient Safety* **33**, 5–14.
27. Entwistle VA (2008) Hurtful comments are harmful comments: respectful communication is not just an optional extra in healthcare. *Health Expectations* **11**, 319–320.
28. Levinson W, Roter DL, Mullooly JP, Dull VT, Frankel RM (1997) Physician-patient communication. The relationship with malpractice claims among primary care physicians and surgeons. *Journal of the American Medical Association* **277**, 553–559.
29. Sorensen R, Iedema R, Piper D, Manias E, Williams A, Tuckett A (2009) Disclosing clinical adverse events to patients: can practice inform policy? *Health Expectations*. Available from: http://www.ncbi.nlm.nih.gov/entrez/query.fcgi?cmd=Retrieve&db=PubMed&dopt=Citation&list_uids=19804555. Accessed: February 23, 2010.
30. Hickson GB, Clayton EW, Githens PB, Sloan FA (1992) Factors that prompted families to file medical malpractice claims following perinatal injuries. *Journal of the American Medical Association* **267**, 1359–1363.
31. Australasian Cochrane Centre (2008) *What Is the Cochrane Library? ACC Guide to the Cochrane Library*. Available from: http://www.cochrane.org.au/libraryguide/guide_whatiscl.php. Accessed: 17 December 2010.

CHAPTER 2

A new conceptual framework for advancing evidence-informed communication and participation

Sophie Hill[1] *and Mary Draper*[2]
[1]Coordinating Editor/Head, Cochrane Consumers and Communication Review Group, Centre for Health Communication and Participation, Australian Institute for Primary Care and Ageing, La Trobe University, Bundoora, Victoria, Australia
[2]Independent Healthcare Consultant, Victoria, Australia

Introduction

It was summer. My (SH) family was having dinner with friends. I was chatting with my host, catching up on the year, and he mentioned he had been to a specialist. The doctor gave him some information about a treatment, which on reflection, sounded too one sided, too 'gung-ho'. Uncertain, he went to another specialist who gave him more information, and they discussed risks and benefits. From the way he told the story, this second approach implied a more cautious path. My friend weighed up the two opinions and opted to go with the second.

This small story is only one experience, but it strikes a chord because we hear many stories like this now. Health consumers – i.e. the knowledgeable patients of the title – are seeking and weighing up health information based on evidence about health treatments, and thinking critically and sceptically about the information they receive in the context of managing their health day to day and communicating with and making decisions with health professionals.

Much – although not all – of the health treatment information which people receive from health professionals is based on evidence [1]. Used in this broader sense, the term 'evidence' could mean several different

The Knowledgeable Patient: Communication and Participation in Health – A Cochrane Handbook, First Edition.
Edited by Sophie Hill.

things. It could mean accumulated clinical experience; it could mean information derived from a new clinical trial; or it could mean information derived from a synthesis of several research studies.

This last meaning is the primary way it is used in this book because the evidence discussed in the chapters that follow is generally evidence presented in a systematic review. Systematic reviews are a type of health research. They have been defined by Sense About Science, a British charitable organisation promoting a better understanding of research, as reports where evidence from a number of studies is gathered together. All available data are pooled and analysed so that the strengths of the evidence can be assessed [2].

Systematic reviews are one of the central pillars of evidence-based healthcare. Evidence-based healthcare originated in the field of medicine [3–7], and has developed into an ethos for wide application in healthcare practice [8], health promotion [9], public health [10, 11] and policy making [12]. Haynes, a leading commentator, has supplied a practical definition of evidence-based medicine as 'a set of tools and resources for finding and applying current best evidence from research for the care of individual patients' [6]. In this context, one of the common meanings of evidence is a systematic review which summarises the results from several clinical trials. This means it refers to evidence about the effects of interventions, where that intervention has been tested in a randomised controlled trial by comparing it with usual care or an alternative to see if the intervention leads to better health outcomes. This is referred to later in this chapter as evidence of effects.

But in telling the opening story, we introduce another element – experience – which can be both collected in research or sought directly from various forms of democratic participation. For instance, research into the social phenomenon of people's experiences can illuminate the meaning of health, the experience of illness or the way in which healthcare happens. This is referred to later as evidence of experiences. These types of understandings may also be sought from individuals with relevant personal or community experience. This book and this chapter are about improving people's health by improving health communication and participation through using and combining these different types of evidence in association with social or civic participation.

The contribution to health of evidence of effects with evidence of experiences, along with democratic participation, is shown in Figure 2.1.

Communication and participation is the central focus

The book places people at its heart and its primary focus is *communication and participation in health*. This term is a shorthand way of referring to a complex set of actions which have meaning and purpose related to

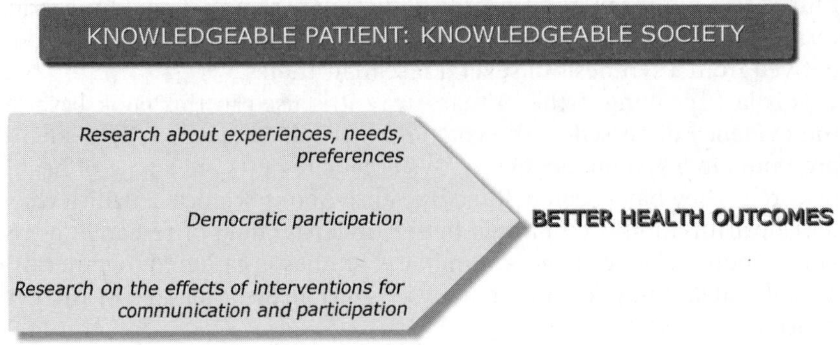

KNOWLEDGEABLE PATIENT: KNOWLEDGEABLE SOCIETY

Research about experiences, needs, preferences

Democratic participation

Research on the effects of interventions for communication and participation

BETTER HEALTH OUTCOMES

Figure 2.1 Knowledgeable patient: knowledgeable society.

improving health. It refers to activities to promote informed and active communication and participation. In practice, this would encompass a wide range of actions seeking patients, health consumers and family carers who are:

- more knowledgeable and competent;
- able to express their views and beliefs;
- making choices alone or with health professionals;
- supported or supportive;
- minimising risks and harms;
- accessing high-quality information and quality health services; and
- participating in policy, research, governance and delivery.

To frame our interests, this chapter advances a new conceptual framework for promoting knowledgeable and confident health consumers and carers, and responsive health systems. We called this 'a conceptual framework for evidence-informed communication and participation'.

The framework is integrative and comprehensive, building on major conceptual frameworks associated with consumer empowerment, patient-centred care and evidence-based healthcare – three key movements for change in health service delivery in the last 30 years. It therefore links science and democracy. The chapter advocates evidence-informed communication and participation as an individual, shared and civic interest. The conceptual framework developed here provides the foundation for the chapters in the book.

What is the broader context?

Consumer empowerment and new policy focus

Over the past 30–40 years, there has been a change in the health landscape, and government policies are increasingly focusing on the role of consumers in the health system. Relevant policy areas cover the full gamut of ways in which individuals and groups intersect with the health system, from member of the public to patient to family carer to community volunteer or advocate. The reasons for this shift are complex and include policies which aim to reduce the cost to government of healthcare (e.g. by preventing illness though a more informed and healthier populace), but also sociopolitical changes associated with having better educated populations, who in turn are seeking to be more in control of their health and lives.

Governments and health organisations are seeking change in the delivery of health services, encouraging services and systems to be more patient- or people centred, so that they can become more responsive to needs [13]. At the same time, there is support across many systems for people to learn the skills to communicate more actively in medical consultations regarding their preferences for treatment [14] or to increase people's skills and capabilities to manage their health, i.e. improve their health literacy [15]. Related to this is the provision of independent information sources for consumers, i.e. sources of information other than via the traditional route of health professionals [16]. Lastly, policies have been introduced to support civic participation in planning and governance [17]. Some international examples of various policies or strategies are provided in Table 2.1, selected to illustrate the different foci of patient-centred or responsive care, active communication and self-management, independent information sources and consumer participation [18].

New roles for consumers, family carers and community members

Active roles

What these policies and initiatives share is a new sense of the role ordinary people can play in healthcare. This role is more commonly an active role and could encompass:

- action taken at different levels, such as at an individual, service or policy-making level [19];
- actions associated with different roles, such as making decisions, managing health, evaluating care and contributing to planning and governance [20].

From patient to consumer: changing terms

In the past, the ordinary person with a stake in the health system was the patient, and the role was largely assumed to be a passive one. With social and political change has come changing terminology. The term commonly used to describe the social agent who adopts these new roles is 'consumer', although language varies with culture and history. More recently, people involved in a caring role – for family, friends or those in the community – have sought to introduce the terms carer, caregiver or peer

Table 2.1 Health policy focus on consumers: selective strategies and policies.

Policy focus	Example of policy or strategy
Patient-centred or responsive care	**People at the Centre of Care Initiative, World Health Organization International Policy Framework** 'Through the biregional People at the Centre of Care Initiative, WHO Western Pacific and South-East Asian regions are adopting a more people-centred and rights-based approach to healthcare in the future work of WHO in the Asia Pacific' The framework identifies four levels of action: **1** individuals, families and communities; **2** health practitioners; **3** healthcare organisations; **4** health systems. www.wpro.who.int/sites/pci/
Active communication and self-management	**'Ask me 3™', USA patient-safety initiative** Developed by the Partnership for Clear Health Communication, National Patient Safety Foundation, Ask Me 3 is a patient education programme designed to promote communication between healthcare providers and patients in order to improve health outcomes. The programme encourages patients to understand the answers to three questions: **1** What is my main problem? **2** What do I need to do? **3** Why is it important for me to do this? www.npsf.org/askme3/ **Healthy Outlook® COPD forecast alert service, UK website and information alert** 'The Met Office has created Healthy Outlook® to help people with COPD take control of their own health and keep well in the winter months.' People with COPD – chronic obstructive pulmonary disease – can opt in to receive a 'recorded voice call by telephone when poor environmental conditions are forecast' www.metoffice.gov.uk/health/public/healthy-outlook.html
Independent information sources	**A–Z in consumer health topics, National Institutes of Health (NIH), USA Department of Health and Human Services** Health information service, linked to sources of reliable information. Editorial policy is that 'NIH health information is based on research results published in peer-reviewed, scientific literature' http://health.nih.gov/

(*Continued*)

Policy focus	Example of policy or strategy
Consumer participation	**Doing it with us not for us: Strategic Direction 2010–2013, Consumer Participation Policy, Victoria, Australia** The policy conceives consumer participation broadly across four levels: **1** individual level, e.g. communicating treatment information; **2** programme or department level, e.g. training staff in communication skills; **3** health service organisation level, e.g. consumer, carer or community member participation in quality programmes; **4** Department of Health level, e.g. providing training to staff on evidence-based participation. www.health.vic.gov.au/consumer/participate.htm

Note: All websites accessed 11 January 2010.

into the political lexicon in response to growing recognition of the role of informal care and its contribution to the health system [21, 22]. Language has been critical to the articulation of needs in the twentieth and twenty-first centuries [23]. To make the case for recognition, groups or individuals need to differentiate themselves from others. There has been debate over the terms used to describe and differentiate consumer roles [24].

In Australia, the term 'consumer' has a sociopolitical meaning (rather than a market or consumerist meaning) and has been used for decades to describe involvement by people in the range of roles described above. Being Australian, we will therefore use it as a critical and conceptually charged term, but we will also use terms such as carers, peers or patients if they fit the context.

Consumers: individual and structured interests

Critical to the formulation of a conceptual approach is the central point that the term 'consumer' refers to someone having diverse interests at different times. Apart from individuals and families with an interest in their personal health, groups of people with a shared interest in health have long been on the health scene, advocating for change. Interests might be social, e.g. the experience of ageing, or it might be their shared experience of a disease. What is different today is the extent to which governments are seeking input from consumers and consumer groups, alongside professional groups, in the formulation of health policy [25]. Consumers are associated with community or consumer groups in several ways: as occasional users of services, as members, and also as members of their governing bodies, influencing new research and services. The role of community groups is being increasingly recognised by governments, possibly because their paid and volunteer services fill gaps in public and private service delivery [26].

Definition and conceptual meaning

In this chapter, we bridge these different roles and levels by using the term *consumer* to conceptually refer to individuals who use health services, but also as a collective term to describe a structured set of interests [27], different from that of health provider and funder interests, and composed of those in roles from patient, to family and community member, to citizen, who all have a stake in a health-producing health system. This adds a civic interest to the role of a consumer as a patient or carer.

So for simplicity, in this chapter we use the term 'consumer' to refer comprehensively to the different roles that people could occupy. In summary, these are:

- as an *individual*, being involved in decisions about one's health, treatment options and management of illness for oneself or someone in the family or community;
- as someone with a *shared* health interest or health condition, working with others to provide information and support to others similarly affected;
- as a citizen and health advocate, being part of and shaping the *civic* dialogue about health and influencing government policy, professional agendas, research, health service delivery and governance.

Common misconceptions

Consumers and communication

Communication is central to thinking about consumers and how to improve healthcare and health outcomes. It is certainly one of the key components of quality for patients and families [28]. A pervasive assumption (or misconception) behind the term 'health communication' is the unidirectional nature of health communication – no doubt deriving historically from the assumption the patient was passive and needed to be informed by a health professional. Chapter 3 takes up this issue in more depth and examines how the multidirectional nature of health communication should be a defining principle of the development of a new shared language for communication interventions.

Here it is sufficient to acknowledge the multidirectional nature of health communication. The implication of this is twofold. First, communication is critical to empowerment because knowing and understanding what is happening, what to do and how to get needed support are central to having control over one's life and health [29]. Second, if communication is multidirectional then consumers are central actors – not peripheral or passive.

Consumers and participation

In health circles, the most common use of the term 'consumer participation' is to mean a lay member of a health service or policy committee, and this use has tended to dominate and obscure the other meanings of the term.

At large, consumer participation can be used to mean a social movement or a strategy to reorient the health system [25]. This sense of the term draws from both its meaning as a form of democratic participation, but also implies sociopolitical change or advocacy.

Consumer participation on working parties, committees or boards is now a common feature of many health systems. For instance, consumers may be involved in working parties to develop clinical practice guidelines. The role of consumer participation is to ensure that issues of importance from a consumer perspective are included and addressed in the guidelines. For instance, in Britain, the National Institute for Health and Clinical Excellence involves consumers and carers in developing guidance and in the stage of implementing it in practice [30]. Frequently, though, consumer participation is used in the minimal sense of gaining some form of feedback from patients [31].

In all these senses, consumer participation has the features of an oral culture, where lived experience and personal testimony are valued [32]. Consumer participation contributes to more responsive and equitable services. It can help to hold health professionals and bureaucrats accountable. It may also reduce political risk in a democratic society, particularly when there is never enough money and always too much demand [31]. And it has the potential to improve health outcomes [33].

Conceptual framework for evidence-informed communication and participation

To overcome the confusion in purpose, context and role, we propose an overarching conceptual framework that integrates the world of multidirectional communication, the world of social participation and knowledge drawn from evidence of experiences and evidence of effects.

A broad foundation is needed for several reasons. We have documented the confusion around different purposes and objects of participation policies. Likewise, communication is a central feature of myriad more focused concepts, such as shared decision-making or patient-centred care. We therefore need a broader foundation which addresses the overall aim of consumer empowerment, but is capable of being specific when required. This helps to disentangle the different purposes which communication and participation might have, depending on the context, people and health issue involved. The framework is also broad enough to capture the centrality of communication and participation to empowerment and health improvement.

Four pillars to empowerment

As an object of social policy, consumer empowerment has been pursued in a range of ways across countries and systems, with some systems adopting all four approaches. These ways can be grouped under four headings, which loosely describe the main focus [28, 34]. Grouped this way, it is therefore possible to see that different strategies to enhance the role and health of consumers may rely on quite different underlying assumptions about their role; for instance, the assumption behind the role of the consumer in a market-oriented strategy is different to the assumption behind a rights-based approach.

The four approaches are as follows:

1. *Scientific approaches,* which rely on empirical research, objective measurement and the systematic gathering of data. The original Pfeffer and Coote model [34] accounted for consumers as subjects, but they are increasingly subjects with agency. Major strategies include researching people's experiences of healthcare in order to improve the quality of care, clinical practice guidelines, systematic reviews and health outcomes research.
2. *Market solutions,* which rely on market information or more responsive services. Consumers are seen as informed choosers in a health market. Information as the basis of choice is the critical strategy. Examples are providing information on service options or performance rankings such as league tables of providers' surgical success or other forms of publication of health service performance.
3. *Legal approaches,* which rely on defined rights or access to judicial and semi-judicial institutions. The assumption is that consumers are citizens with rights. Strategies include health charters, legislation to protect consumers' interests, the role of informed consent, and the right and opportunity to make a complaint.
4. *Democratic participation,* which relies on ways to participate individually or collectively in health decisions. Consumers are seen as equal partners and citizens. Main strategies would include websites providing health and treatment information which informs decision-making, promoting models for shared decision-making and consumer participation in decision-making structures.

A robust approach to consumer empowerment might adopt strategies from each approach and be clear about the assumptions at play. For example, while publication of health service performance was initially thought to be a market strategy affecting consumer choice, its usefulness from a consumer perspective is more about transparency and accountability – democratic participation [35].

Combining scientific approaches and democratic participation

The overarching and integrated conceptual framework advanced here rests on the twin pillars of scientific approaches and democratic participation. This assumes that neither alone is sufficient, but used together, they contribute more powerfully to improving health and health services.

Democratic (individual) participation on a committee can contribute useful information about consumer experiences, but is powerfully aided by learning from previous research about the breadth of people's health experiences and from evaluations from a consumer perspective. Certainly, consumer participation should be woven through research – informing its formulation, aiding its conduct and influencing how it is adopted. But more importantly, democratic participation should be seen as a strategy working in conjunction with scientific approaches for improving health.

This is captured in Figure 2.2. This shows that at all stages of health policy and service improvement, *scientific approaches* (i.e. learning from research from different types of studies) and *democracy* (through consumer participation by consumers and carers) could improve the decision-making process. The process is cyclical, recognising that new problems may emerge following change. See Graham et al., 2006, 'Lost in knowledge translation: time for a map?' for a more detailed map of the processes to address the knowledge to action gap [36]. The central role of evaluation and monitoring to consumer participation is captured in the Australian consumer participation policy for the state of Victoria [18].

The importance of combining scientific approaches with democratic participation underpins new initiatives such as the James Lind Alliance

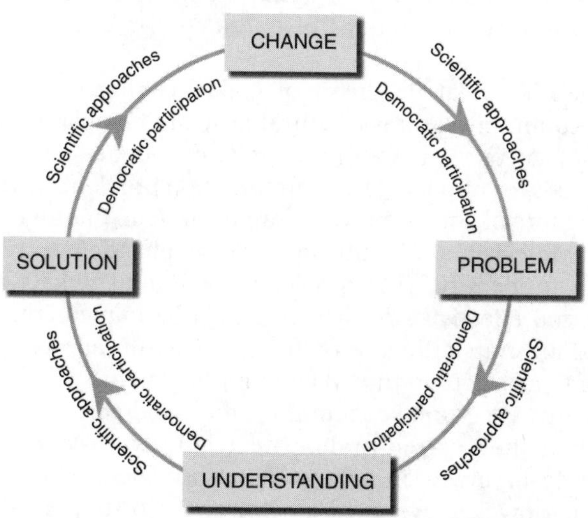

Figure 2.2 Contribution of science and democracy to health service improvement.

[37]. This is a non-profit initiative, based in England but with an international scope, which brings together consumers and health professionals to identify those questions which have not been answered by health research and to set priorities for new research.

Similarly, the international organisation The Cochrane Collaboration, which publishes systematic reviews of the effects of interventions, is formed around principles of rigorous science and participation [38]. It has an organisational structure which combines participation by many different health professional groups, researchers and consumers to produce research syntheses or systematic reviews of the evidence of effects [39].

Cochrane review groups which address issues identified by consumers, and the Cochrane Consumers and Communication Review Group [40] – focusing as it does on interventions affecting people's interactions with the health system – increasingly bring evidence to complement the lived experience of consumers. Evidence in systematic reviews, assembled, quality assessed and synthesised for future decision-making, is an efficient use of the public resource of past research [41].

Conclusion: advancing evidence-informed communication and participation

This leads us to five concluding remarks:

1 Integrating scientific approaches (e.g. evidence-based healthcare and systematic reviews) with democratic participation (e.g. individual or civic involvement) leads to awareness that not only should recommended health treatments be based where possible on rigorous evidence of benefit, but approaches to communicating with and involving people should also be based where possible on evidence of effectiveness. This is the basis of *evidence-informed communication and participation*.

2 Communication is at the heart of good healthcare; this is the reason why communication is a central factor in complaints and adverse events [42]. A consequence of focusing on evidence for effective communication is to shift debate and attention on problems with the health system to more of a focus on what can be done to improve it. Adopting the twin strategies of scientific approaches plus democratic participation helps to identify what problems are serious, what solutions are available and effective, and which should be implemented and how. Figure 2.2 illustrated the intertwining of scientific approaches and participation to all stages in the cycle of improvement.

3 Governments need to take communication and participation more seriously than they currently do. The relatively easy option for governments is to invest in information strategies, which is certainly important. However, we need governments to support and invest in strategies that enable – not just inform. This will take investment.

Community groups, working to improve the care of women with breast cancer, have led the way: witness, for example, the investment in evidence and information to bring women into a partnership around treatments for breast cancer [43]. This issue has particular relevance for strategies to bring individual, shared or civic interests into the ambit of evidence-based healthcare, because this domain has traditionally been dominated by the voices and interests of health professionals and researchers.

4 Government involvement is essential in taking the lead on actions to reduce health inequities, to look across services and domains to see who is missing out on the benefits of a healthy life and access to necessary and responsive services. Improving health generally may not lead to fair health benefits for all. People with poorer health literacy, for example, do not fare as well in terms of health status and health outcomes [44]. For this reason, the Final Report to the World Health Organization on the *Social Determinants of Health* in 2007 recommended that 'actions to tackle the social determinants of poor health and health inequities must focus on the causes of health inequities rather than general health improvement' [45].

5 The fifth issue is one about systems. Examine the issue of decision aids – shown to be effective for various decision-making outcomes in a review of 55 randomised controlled trials [46, 47]. Subject to local need and circumstances, how do the findings of this review get implemented? It is not just about a few individuals making a change. Rather it would require systems to change, e.g. support at an institutional level, professional training and development, clinical, consumer and epidemiological research input to the decision aid itself, changes to procedures, patient involvement and education, and so on. This implies that evidence for improving communication and participation has to be embedded in new models of care. Similarly, evidence in systematic reviews for improving communication, drawn from studies with people with various health problems, can inform the processes and systems for improving the delivery of evidence-based clinical care.

This chapter has been about the nexus of science and democracy in health and how an approach which combines these domains can be harnessed to improve health outcomes. Evidence-informed communication and participation is an individual, shared and civic interest. The framework proposed here asserts the centrality of communication and participation to improved health and provides the foundation for the chapters in the book.

References

1. Buchan H, Sewell JR, Sweet M (2004) Translating evidence into practice. *The Medical Journal of Australia* **180**, S43.

2. Sense About Science (2009) *Systematic Reviews*. Available from: http://www.senseaboutscience.org.uk/PDF/SenseAboutSystematicReviews.pdf. Accessed: 7 July 2010.
3. Evidence-Based Medicine Working Group, Gordon Guyatt et al. (1992) Evidence-based medicine: a new approach to teaching the practice of medicine. *Journal of the American Medical Association* **268**, 2420–2425.
4. Rosenberg W, Donald A (1995) Evidence based medicine: an approach to clinical problem-solving. *British Medical Journal* **310**, 1122–1126.
5. Sackett DL, Rosenberg WMC, Gray JAM, Haynes RB, Richardson WS (1996) Evidence based medicine: what it is and what it isn't. *British Medical Journal* **312**, 71–72.
6. Haynes RB (2002) What kind of evidence is it that evidence-based medicine advocates want health care providers and consumers to pay attention to? *BMC Health Services Research* **2**, 3.
7. Daly J (2005) *Evidence-Based Medicine and the Search for a Science of Clinical Care*. University of California Press, California.
8. Dawes M, Summerskill W, Glasziou P, et al. (2005) Sicily statement on evidence-based practice. *BMC Medical Education* **5**, 1.
9. Oliver S, Peersman G (2002) *Using Research for Effective Health Promotion*. Open University Press, Buckingham.
10. Petticrew M, Roberts H (2006) *Systematic Reviews in the Social Sciences*. Blackwell Publishing, Malden.
11. Brownson RC, Fielding JE, Maylahn CM (2009) Evidence-based public health: a fundamental concept for public health practice. *Annual Review of Public Health* **30**, 175–201.
12. Lin V, Gibson B (2003) *Evidence-Based Health Policy*. Oxford University Press, South Melbourne.
13. World Health Organization, South East Asian Region, Western Pacific Region (2007) *People at the Centre of Health Care. Harmonizing Mind and Body, People and Systems*. World Health Organization. Available from: http://www.wpro.who.int/publications/PUB_139789290613169.htm. Accessed: 19 February 2010.
14. Edwards A, Elwyn G (2009) *Shared Decision-Making in Health Care: Achieving Evidence-Based Patient Choice*. Oxford University Press, Oxford.
15. Nutbeam D (2000) Health literacy as a public health goal: a challenge for contemporary health education and communication strategies into the 21st century. *Health Promotion International* **15**, 259–267.
16. Hill S (2003) What is new in health information? Evidence for consumers and policy making. In: Lin V, Gibson B, (eds.) *Evidence-Based Health Policy: Problems and Possibilities*. Oxford University Press, Melbourne.
17. Court J, Mendizabal E, Osborne D, Young J (2006) *Policy Engagement: How Civil Society Can Be More Effective*. Overseas Development Institute, London.
18. Victorian Government (2009) *Doing It With Us Not for Us: Strategic Direction 2010–13*. Rural and Regional Health and Aged Care Services Division Victorian Government Department of Health, Melbourne. Available from: http://www.health.vic.gov.au/consumer/downloads/strategic_direction_2010-13.pdf. Accessed: 18 February 2010.
19. Crawford MJ, Rutter D, Manley C, et al. (2002) Systematic review of involving patients in the planning and development of health care. *British Medical Journal* **325**, 1263.

20. Coulter A (2002) *The Autonomous Patient: Ending Paternalism in Medical Care*. The Nuffield Trust, London.
21. Carers Australia (2009) Submission to the National Human Rights Consultation, Australia, June 2009. Available from: http://www.carersaustralia.com.au/?/national/section/14:policy-work/1. Accessed: 2 June 2010.
22. UK Department of Health (2008) *Carers at the Heart of 21st-Century Families and Communities*. HM Government, England. Available from: http://www.dh.gov.uk/en/publicationsandstatistics/publications/publicationspolicyandguidance/dh_085345. Accessed: 2 June 2010.
23. Fraser N (1989) Struggle over needs: outline of a socialist-feminist critical theory of late capitalist political culture. *Unruly Practices: Power, Discourse and Gender in Contemporary Social Theory*. Polity Press, Cambridge, pp. 161–187.
24. Herxheimer A, Goodare H (1999) Who are you, and who are we? Looking through some key words. *Health Expectations* **2**, 3–6.
25. Baggott R, Allsop J, Jones K (2005) *Speaking for Patients and Carers: Health Consumer Groups and the Policy Process*. Palgrave MacMillan, Hampshire and New York.
26. Australian Government (2010) *National Compact: Working Together*. Available from: http://www.nationalcompact.gov.au/wordpress/wp-content/uploads/Nat_compact.pdf. Accessed: 3 June 2010.
27. Duckett SJ (1984) Structural interests and Australian health policy. *Social Science & Medicine* **18**, 959–966.
28. Draper M, Hill S (1996) *The Role of Patient Satisfaction Surveys in a National Approach to Hospital Quality Management*. Australian Government Publishing Service, Canberra. Available from: www.healthissuescentre.org.au/documents/detail.chtml?filename_num=226730. Accessed: 12 January 2010.
29. Segal L (1998) The importance of patient empowerment in health system reform. *Health Policy* **44**, 31–44.
30. National Institute for Health and Clinical Excellence (2010) *Patient and Public Involvement*. Available from: http://www.nice.org.uk/getinvolved/patientandpublicinvolvement/patient_and_public_involvement.jsp. Accessed: 7 June 2010.
31. Horey D, Hill S (2005) *Engaging Consumers in Health Policy. 3rd AIHPS Health Policy Roundtable*. Parliament House Canberra, 8 November 2005. Available from: http://www.aihps.org/component/option,com_docman/task,cat_view/gid,65/dir,DESC/order,name/limit,5/limitstart,5/. Accessed: 12 January 2010.
32. Hill S (2005) *Why Should We Evaluate Consumer Participation? Learning From Our Experience and the Evidence*. Paper to the Researching Consumer Participation Symposium. Organised by the Cochrane Consumers and Communication Review Group and the Victorian Department of Human Services Quality Branch, Melbourne.
33. Nilsen ES, Myrhaug HT, Johansen M, Oliver S, Oxman AD (2006) Methods of consumer involvement in developing healthcare policy and research, clinical practice guidelines and patient information material. *Cochrane Database of Systematic Reviews*, CD004563.
34. Pfeffer N, Coote A (1991) *Is Quality Good for You?* Institute for Public Policy Research, London.
35. Marshall MN, Shekelle PG, Davies HTO, Smith PC (2003) Public reporting on quality in the United States and the United Kingdom. *Health Affairs* **22**, 134–148.

36. Graham ID, Logan J, Harrison MB, et al. (2006) Lost in knowledge translation: time for a map? *The Journal of Continuing Education in the Health Professions* **26**, 13–24.
37. Chalmers I (2010) Systematic reviews and uncertainties about the effects of treatments [editorial]. *The Cochrane Library.* Available from: http://www.thecochranelibrary.com/details/editorial/691951/Systematic-reviews-and-uncertainties-about-the-effects-of-treatments-by-Sir-Iain.html. Accessed: 26 August 2010.
38. The Cochrane Collaboration (2010) *Ten Key Principles.* Available from: http://www.cochrane.org/about-us/our-principles. Accessed: 26 August 2010.
39. The Cochrane Collaboration (2004) *Newcomers' Guide to the Cochrane Collaboration.* Available from: http://www2.cochrane.org/docs/newcomers_guide_paper_0205.doc. Accessed: 26 August 2010.
40. Prictor M, Hill S, Car J, et al. (2010) Cochrane Consumers and Communication Group. *About the Cochrane Collaboration (Cochrane Review Groups (CRGs)),* Issue 1. Art. no.: COMMUN.
41. Light R, Pillemer D (1984) *Summing up*. Harvard University Press, Cambridge.
42. Office of the Health Services Commissioner (2009) *Office of the Health Services Commissioner, Annual Report 2009.* Department of Health Victoria, Melbourne. Available from: http://www.health.vic.gov.au/hsc/resources/annualrep.htm. Accessed: 1 June 2010.
43. Australia. National Breast and Ovarian Cancer Centre (2009) Who's who in breast cancer? Available from: http://www.nbocc.org.au/our-organisation/about-nbocc/national-breast-cancer-organisations. Accessed: 10 June 2010.
44. US Department of Health and Human Services, Office of Disease Prevention and Health Promotion (n.d.) *Fact Sheet: Health Literacy and Health Outcomes.* USA Office of Disease Prevention and Health Promotion. Available from: http://www.health.gov/communication/literacy/quickguide/factsliteracy.htm. Accessed: 26 August 2010.
45. Kelly MP, Morgan A, Bonnefoy J, Butt J, Bergman V (2007) *The Social Determinants of Health: Developing an Evidence Base for Political Action. Final Report to the World Health Organization Commission on the Social Determinants of Health.* Universidad del Desarrollo, Chile and National Institute for Health and Clinical Excellence, United Kingdom. Available from: http://www.who.int/social_determinants/resources/mekn_final_report_102007.pdf. Accessed: 25 August 2010.
46. O'Connor AM, Bennett CL, Stacey D, et al. (2009) Decision aids for people facing health treatment or screening decisions. *Cochrane Database of Systematic Reviews,* CD001431.
47. Légaré F, Ratté S, Stacey D, et al. (2010) Interventions for improving the adoption of shared decision making by healthcare professionals. *Cochrane Database of Systematic Reviews,* CD006732.

CHAPTER 3

Interventions for communication and participation: their purpose and practice

Sophie Hill[1], *Dianne B. Lowe*[2] *and Rebecca E. Ryan*[3]
[1]Coordinating Editor/Head, Cochrane Consumers and Communication Review Group, Centre for Health Communication and Participation, Australian Institute for Primary Care and Ageing, La Trobe University, Bundoora, Victoria, Australia
[2]Research Officer, Cochrane Consumers and Communication Review Group, Centre for Health Communication and Participation, Australian Institute for Primary Care and Ageing, La Trobe University, Bundoora, Victoria, Australia
[3]Research Fellow, Cochrane Consumers and Communication Review Group, Centre for Health Communication and Participation, Australian Institute for Primary Care and Ageing, La Trobe University, Bundoora, Victoria, Australia

Any way you look at it, communication and participation are integral to health improvement, health policy and service delivery. All actions to provide health treatment involve an act of communication with the intended recipient, whether to a member of the public or a patient in the consulting room. Every aspect of how an individual manages their health draws from information received and interactions with others at many different levels, from family to society.

In Chapter 2, an overarching conceptual framework was outlined, which advanced the argument for using scientific approaches (using knowledge derived from research, including systematic reviews) with democratic participation (i.e. consumers having a structured interest around individual, shared and civic roles). This begs the question: if we wish to advance evidence-informed communication and participation, what do we mean by *interventions* for communication and participation?

The Knowledgeable Patient: Communication and Participation in Health – A Cochrane Handbook, First Edition. Edited by Sophie Hill.

This chapter defines interventions for communication and participation. It outlines the special features of interventions for communication and participation in a way that is holistic (helping to understand and relate parts to a complex whole), but also practical and particularistic. This may aid the development of a shared language to discuss our intentions and the interventions we select to achieve these aims. This can lead to examining, through research, whether our aims are met or not – covered in Chapter 4. A case study of communication for safe medicine use will provide a practical demonstration of how to expand our notions of communication and participation through the construction of a new taxonomy of interventions. Lastly, new thinking around evaluating social processes and complexity and the involvement of consumers in developing interventions is highlighted.

What are interventions?

Communication and participation are like air. We are part of them; they are part of us. Communication and the processes of being involved are so pervasive and intrinsic to social life and to healthcare that it is difficult to break them down into specific actions.

Yet not every act of communication is the same. To illustrate, let us take a new concept and practice called 'personalised risk communication'. A general practitioner (GP) and a 55-year-old woman are engaged in a medical consultation for a general health check-up. The woman smokes and would like to give up. The GP, drawing from national guidelines for preventing cardiovascular disease, shows the woman a graph which indicates she is at high risk of heart disease (an absolute risk of 1 in 6) and that her heart could be viewed as the same as a woman who is 67 [1].

This act of communication is an intervention. It is called personalised risk communication. It is called *risk communication* because the risk for heart disease has been calculated from large epidemiological studies, quantified and presented in a visual format for communication with patients. It is termed *personalised* because the epidemiological data on the incidence of heart disease associated with specific risks has been transformed into a risk for women of a specific age group, risk factors and health status (in this case woman, aged 55, who smokes and is therefore at risk for heart disease). The GP has alternatives to personalised risk. She or he could simply talk about the dangers of smoking in general – or mention risk for heart disease but not calculate a specific risk relevant to the individual patient.

What makes personalised risk – the example used here – an intervention?

In public health, a field highly relevant to communication and participation, we find a definition of interventions as follows: 'an intervention comprises an action or programme to bring about identifiable outcomes

[2]'. This definition makes the connection between purposeful actions and the outcomes that are sought, but it does not deal with the invisibility of communication and participation. To address this we need to articulate the features of interventions.

Features of interventions for communication and participation

To establish a definition which is comprehensive but practical, we need to tease out the features of interventions for communication and participation, working through three steps and using the personalised risk communication example to illustrate each step and component.

Step 1: To be an intervention for communication and participation, it should have the following major features:

- *Purposeful, with a clear aim:* Communication to reduce risk for heart disease.
- *Planned:* GP intends to use personalised risk communication in every applicable instance with patients in consultations, in line with advice from best practice clinical guidelines.
- *Formalised:* This is the basics, the 'what', 'who', 'where', 'how' and 'when' of interventions [3]. Specifically, the communication has *core content* (epidemiological evidence and quantified risk levels transformed into an absolute risk figure). The *mode of delivery* is verbal plus visual information. There is an explicit or designated *format* for the visual risk (bar chart with comparative information). The *parties involved* in the communication exchange are the GP (responsible for initiating risk communication) and the patient. The *timing* and *context* for this intervention are in a consultation for a general health check-up.

Step 2: Interventions for communication and participation have the potential for added features. These are associated with responding to the contextual complexity of communication and the variable nature of people's needs:

- *Repeatable:* The GP can repeat the communication for all relevant patients or with the same patient over time.
- *Sequenced or timed:* The GP can introduce the concept and information at different stages of a consultation or at different points in the patient's medical encounters.
- *Modifiable:* The risk calculation tool provides absolute risks for people of different ages and risk levels. It can be personalised or tailored [4]. It can be modified for use by different parties in variable settings, for example, by community nurses or specialists or by consumers via the internet.
- *Adaptable:* The risk communication information can be produced in different formats (e.g. take-home information), can have different levels of reading accessibility or can be translated into community languages.

- *It can be combined:* The single-risk communication message can be delivered on its own or combined with other interventions, e.g. counselling to quit smoking.
- *Classifiable:* As a class or category of communication tasks, it can be defined and described. Its classification may be linked to the theory which has informed its development, for instance, theories on behaviour change [5] associated with understanding and responding to risk information.

Step 3: In the context of evidence-informed communication and participation, the evidence for the effects (benefits or harms) of interventions can be demonstrated and accumulated:

- *Effects evaluated rigorously:* The effects of personalised risk communication [6] on various outcomes (e.g. knowledge of risk and changes in risky behaviour) can be assessed by conducting a randomised controlled trial (RCT), a rigorous way of evaluating the effects of interventions on health outcomes. In the trial, patients are randomised either to an intervention group, where GPs deliver personalised risk communication, or to a control group, where GPs communicate risk in general terms. After a set period of time, the outcomes for both the groups are measured and compared to see if personalised risk communication is more effective than the comparator for the desired outcome.
- *Evidence for decision-makers synthesised:* The evidence on the effects of more than one RCT can be summarised in a systematic review to give an overall assessment of the evidence from all available and relevant trials: see an example in the Cochrane systematic review on 'Personalised risk communication for informed decision-making about taking screening tests' by Edwards and colleagues [7].

In summary, an intervention for communication and participation can be defined as a purposeful, planned and formalised strategy associated with a diverse range of intentions or aims, including to inform, educate, communicate with, support, skill, change behaviour, engage and seek participation of people in all spheres of health from individual to collective contexts. An intervention, depending on the context and needs of communication or participation, can be repeated, sequenced, modified or adapted as required. It may be combined with other intervention elements and classified for analysis and knowledge transfer. Evidence on its effects can be derived and accumulated.

Principles for interventions for communication and participation

In Chapter 2, the centrality of consumers and carers to the social processes of communication and participation was stated. This is conceptually linked to the principle of recognising the multidirectional [8] nature of communication and participation. The opposite of multidirectional communication would be unidirectional communication. In fact, reading many news articles about health can make you feel that communication is mainly unidirectional, i.e. to consumers. People are usually presented as the recipients of information and communication, such as advice on what to do to keep healthy, get screened, take up needed healthcare and so on. The importance of information coming from consumers or the reality of many consumers communicating with each other does not receive the same attention.

Analysis of thousands of interventions for communication and participation in fact identifies that communication and participation can be readily conceived as multidirectional. The Cochrane Consumers and Communication Review Group has analysed its Trials Register to assess and code the number of interventions in trials according to six broad communication directions. The six directions were:

1 interventions directed to the consumer;
2 interventions from the consumer;
3 interventions for communication exchange between health providers and consumers;
4 interventions for communication between consumers;
5 interventions for communication to the healthcare provider from another source;
6 service delivery and policy interventions.

This way of breaking down communication not only recognises the centrality of consumers to healthcare, but also posits consumers as providers of valid information. Consumers are therefore legitimate and potentially authoritative sources – of information about their symptoms or experiences and of input to decision-making about preferences for treatments or values about desired health states. This perspective can be reflected in the movement to build patient-reported outcomes [9,10]: this is discussed further in Chapter 4.

The analysis was conducted on 6728 trials, selected from Issue 3, 2007, of the Central Register of Controlled Trials in *The Cochrane Library*. Results are presented in Table 3.1 as a number and percentage of the total. The results do not add to 100% because multifaceted interventions may be coded for more than one direction of communication. It should not be assumed that some categories have the sum of all the trials in the area. For instance, the Cochrane Effective Practice and Organisation of Care (EPOC) review group has a register of trials relevant to their scope of work and this will contain many trials of service interventions. However, the Consumers and Communication Register has been developed from searching for, screening and selecting trials relevant to communication and participation, and is therefore is a reliable epidemiological snapshot of what has been researched.

Coding and analysis according to the principal direction of communication highlight immediately that the unidirectional approach – whilst dominant – is not a complete reflection of the complexity of interventions in this domain of health.

Table 3.1 Direction of communication and participation interventions.

Interventions by main direction of communication, with intervention examples	No. of trials	Expressed as % of 6728 trials
1 Interventions directed to the consumer, e.g. medicine instruction and patient education	5218	78
2 Interventions from the consumer, e.g. patient reporting of self-monitoring and patient profiling	1364	20
3 Interventions for communication exchange between health providers and consumers, e.g. decision aid and goal setting	1965	29
4 Interventions for communication between consumers, e.g. self-help group and family teamwork	986	15
5 Interventions for communication to the healthcare provider from another source, e.g. communication skills training and clinician reminder system	182	3
6 Service delivery and policy interventions, e.g. family access and choice of health, professional	783	12

Building knowledge in a field of social complexity

Communication is a complex social process that involves the exchange of both information and meaning [11]. While there are different theoretical approaches to communication, it is commonly acknowledged that, in addition to the characteristics of the communication process (e.g. Rimal and Lapinski, 2009, list 'channel, source, receiver and message'), understandings of information are socially mediated at both individual and societal levels and there is a process of social interaction, exchange and creation of meaning [12].

The principle of multidirectional communication takes this one step further because it acknowledges the role of consumers as key communicators, originating communication as well as the recipients of communications. Consumers are therefore creating new meanings for health, and this can be witnessed through the use of social media [13].

What distinguishes the approach described here is the emphasis on interventions for purposeful communication and participation associated with a diversity of health-related aims. In this approach, an intervention could be a person who communicates a specific message, two or more people in an exchange, a website with interactivity, a group of people providing support or a health service involving community members in planning. Interventions are therefore not defined by the specific delivery mechanism or by the act of communication per se, but by the intention to bring about better health through diverse interactive and purposeful means. This complexity – and consequent opportunity for confusion from language and meaning – raises the need for a knowledge tool, or taxonomy.

The development of taxonomies of interventions

Associated with evidence-based healthcare has been the development of taxonomies of interventions. A taxonomy is a classification scheme which organises phenomena – in this case, interventions – on the basis of conceptual or practical similarities. The need to develop taxonomies is associated with the knowledge production processes of building evidence [14]. Taxonomies help in different ways. They help to overcome the confusion of language and meaning, i.e. where different terms have been used for the same action or different actions. They help to group intervention types into logical groups or categories. This can aid future research, but also knowledge transfer, the process of promoting the adoption of evidence in practice [15,16] (see Chapter 17). As a tool, they can be used to show where evidence has been assembled and summarised and where gaps in knowledge exist.

Intervention features explained earlier are critical to the development of taxonomic categories. An ideal intervention should be purposeful, planned and formalised, related to the overarching concept of *intentional action*, affecting others and with effects that can be measured. This overarching concept informs the development of evidence-based taxonomies or taxonomies for informing or organising evidence. Second, an intervention being repeatable, sequenced, modifiable, adaptable, etc., implies that a different array of interventions could meet the aims or intentions of a taxonomic category. For instance, the aim of teaching skills could be done using face-to-face interventions or via the internet.

A taxonomy of interventions for communication and participation about medicines

This thinking led to the development of a taxonomy of consumer-oriented interventions to improve the use of medicines [17]. The taxonomy is used to organise concise summaries of review-level evidence in a Canadian database called *Rx for Change*, found at: http://www.cadth.ca/index.php/en/compus/optimal-ther-resources/interventions. The database is a joint collaboration of the Canadian Optimal Medication Prescribing and Utilization Service (COMPUS), the Cochrane Effective Practice and Organisation of Care and the Cochrane Consumers and Communication Review Groups [18].

The database houses evidence to aid knowledge transfer for improving the way in which medicines are prescribed and taken. The range of strategies or interventions considered by the database include those directed principally to health professionals and services, such as regulatory strategies, education or interventions to improve the way in which healthcare is organised, and those termed consumer oriented, including a broad range of strategies to affect the ways people interact and manage their medicines.

One of the challenges for organising review-level evidence has been the historically oriented focus on adherence by the patient to take their medicines 'as directed' [19]. This focus has come under increasing criticism for social and health-related reasons. The development of a new taxonomy had to take into account the multidirectionality of communication, diversity of interventions potentially applicable and comprehensive range of purposes associated with improving medicine use.

The taxonomy was developed by analysing thematically the existing definitions of simple and complex interventions to improve prescribing and medicines use behaviours which were aimed at consumers either directly (e.g. patient education) or indirectly (e.g. communication skills training for doctors). In total, eight recurrent themes were identified from the interventions analysed, and these formed the basis of the intervention categories. The definition of each category and examples of specific interventions within each are outlined in Table 3.2.

The complexity of potential choices facing health professionals is demonstrated by overlap between taxonomy categories. Interventions (particularly multifaceted interventions) may fit within more than one category, depending on the purpose of the intervention. For example, a complex intervention aiming to improve medicines adherence may include provision of education sessions, case managers and reminders, and so may map to the following taxonomy categories:

- providing information and education (education sessions);
- improving quality (case managers); and
- supporting behaviour change (reminders).

This means that while taxonomies aid clear thinking about complex interventions, the key issue is to examine the main purposes of the intervention, as this indicates the outcomes that are ultimately sought.

New insights into complex interventions

As evidence-based healthcare has developed over time, the methods for conducting systematic reviews have spread in application, with more complex interventions increasingly becoming the subject of trials and therefore reviews. This leads to challenges in conducting research and interpreting evidence.

What are complex interventions? Complexity can be examined from several standpoints: Craig and colleagues identify the multiple factors such as the number of interacting components, the number or difficulty of behaviours, the groups or levels targeted, the range of outcomes sought and the degree of modification [20]. These criteria would apply to most of the interventions for communication and participation.

Table 3.2 Taxonomy of interventions for consumers' medicines use.

Taxonomic categories and definition	Examples of interventions
To inform and educate Strategies to enable consumers to know about their treatment and their health. Interventions include those to educate, to inform or to promote health or treatment. Interventions can be provided to individuals or groups, in print or verbally, or face to face or remotely. Interventions may be simple or complex, such as those to manage health or treatment as part of a multifaceted strategy	• Written medicines information, e.g. fact sheets • Patient information materials, e.g. booklets and videos • Generic or tailored education • Visual aids • Advertising campaigns
To support behaviour change Strategies focusing on the adoption or promotion of health and treatment behaviours, such as adherence to medicines. Interventions may address behaviour change for the underuse, overuse or misuse of medicines, and may include practical strategies to assist consumers in taking their medicines correctly	• Reminder devices, e.g. alarms or pill boxes • Patient reminders or recall systems, e.g. postcards • Patient diaries • Simplified dose or frequency • Pharmacist-led services • Feedback on clinical markers
To teach skills Strategies focusing on the acquisition of skills relevant to medicines use. Interventions aim to assist consumers to develop a broad set of competencies around medicines use and health, such as medicines management, or training consumers in the correct use of treatments or devices to deliver treatment	• Training sessions • Self-management medicines programmes • Problem-solving skills training • Self-monitoring, with or without self-adjustment
To facilitate communication and/or decision-making Strategies to involve consumers in decision-making about medicines. Interventions include those that aim to help consumers make decisions about medicines, such as interventions to encourage expression of their values or preferences, and/or to optimise communication with consumers about medicines	• Decision aids • Communication skills training for clinicians and/or patients • Written action plans • Written question lists for pharmacists
To support Strategies to provide assistance and encouragement to help consumers cope with and manage their health and related medicines use. Interventions can target patients or carers, as individuals or in groups, and may be delivered face to face or remotely	• Counselling (in many forms) • Therapy, e.g. cognitive behavioural therapy • Peer support programmes • Crisis interventions

(Continued)

Table 3.2 *(Continued)*

Taxonomic categories and definition	Examples of interventions
To minimise risks and harms Strategies specifically focusing on preventing or managing adverse events of treatment and complications of disease. Interventions can be for ongoing treatment or related to emergency events. Strategies aim to minimise risks or harms at an individual or a population level, such as reducing antibiotic use or augmenting immunisation uptake	• Consumer reporting of adverse events • Mass mailings for immunisation uptake, e.g. personalised letters • Medicines review to reduce adverse events such as falls • Using patient's own medicines in hospital setting
To involve consumers at the systems level Strategies to involve consumers in decision-making processes on medicines prescribing and use at a system level, such as in research planning, formulary and policy decisions. Interventions can involve consumers in different roles, such as planning, research, audit and review, and governance	• Guideline committee involvement • Peer review for research • Involvement in development of patient medicines information
To improve healthcare quality Strategies to improve the total package, coordination or integration of care delivered. Interventions can involve substitution or expansion of one type of care, such as interventions that aim to overcome system barriers to medicines use, including access and financial barriers	• Pharmaceutical care plan and follow-up • Pharmacist–GP liaison • Financial incentives, co-payments or formulary interventions, e.g. generic substitution • Decision support systems

Adapted with permission of Elsevier from Lowe D, Ryan R, Santesso N, Hill S (In press) Development of a taxonomy of interventions to organise the evidence on consumers' medicines use. *Patient Education and Counseling.* doi:10.1016/j.pec.2010.09.024. Copyright © 2010, Elsevier Publishing.

Complex interventions throw up many challenges. Michie and colleagues have argued that developing new interventions should take account of the theoretical basis for linking the intervention purpose to the outcomes which are sought [5]. Systematic reviews should address this similarly by documenting the theoretical basis of interventions in trials and analysing the effects with this in mind. Shepperd and colleagues [21] write that the lack of agreed definitions hinders both the production and the use of evidence. Their solutions to this problem include developing typologies (such as the taxonomy described above) and gathering supplementary information to aid both evidence synthesis and knowledge transfer. Finally, Glasziou and colleagues [3] advance a range of strategies to improve both understanding of interventions and their evidence-based use in practice. These include involving end-users in developing interventions and improving the description of interventions in documents or registers which identify and summarise the research undertaken in controlled trials and systematic reviews.

Involving consumers in the development of interventions has taken a step forward through programmes such as the Australian programme in Victoria, titled 'Evaluating the Effectiveness of Participation' (discussed further in Chapter 17). Funding for evaluating consumer participation interventions is in part conditional on the health service involving consumers in the development or delivery of the intervention. Similarly, the Cochrane Consumers and Communication Review Group encourages authors of systematic reviews to collect information about whether consumers or carers have been involved in the design of the intervention [22]. For example, Ryan and co-authors conducted a systematic review of audio-visual presentation of information for informed consent for participation in clinical trials and checked all the included trials to see if consumers were involved in the development of the intervention [23]. Of the four trials providing data for the review, only one had involved consumers. This was a trial to evaluate the effect of a patient information video during the informed consent process of a perinatal trial, and in this case, actual patients were involved in the production of the video intervention [24].

This chapter has outlined the features of interventions for communication and participation, highlighting the importance of intention or purpose. The complexity of those purposes notwithstanding, researchers are seeking to establish what the effects are of deliberate, purposeful communication or participation strategies. This is the subject of the next chapter.

References

1. Hill S, Spink J, Cadilhac D, et al. (2010) Absolute risk representation in cardiovascular disease prevention: comprehension and preferences of healthcare consumers and general practitioners involved in a focus group study. *BMC Public Health* **10**, 108.
2. Rychetnik L, Hawe P, Waters E, Barratt A, Frommer M (2004) A glossary for evidence based public health. *Journal of Epidemiology and Community Health* **58**, 538–545.
3. Glasziou P, Chalmers I, Altman DG, et al. (2010) Taking healthcare interventions from trial to practice. *British Medical Journal* **341**, c3852.
4. Lustria ML, Cortese J, Noar SM, Glueckauf RL (2009) Computer-tailored health interventions delivered over the Web: review and analysis of key components. *Patient Education and Counseling* **74**, 156–173.
5. Michie S, Fixsen D, Grimshaw JM, Eccles MP (2009) Specifying and reporting complex behaviour change interventions: the need for a scientific method. *Implementation Science* **4**, 40.

6. Edwards A, Thomas R, Williams R, Ellner AL, Brown P, Elwyn G (2006) Presenting risk information to people with diabetes: evaluating effects and preferences for different formats by a web-based randomised controlled trial. *Patient Education and Counseling* **63**, 336–349.
7. Edwards AG, Evans R, Dundon J, Haigh S, Hood K, Elwyn GJ (2006) Personalised risk communication for informed decision making about taking screening tests. *Cochrane Database of Systematic Reviews*, CD001865.
8. Hill S (2009) Directions in health communication. *Bulletin of the World Health Organization* **87**, 648.
9. PatientView (2008) *Outcomes in Clinical Research – Whose Responsibility?* Report of a Seminar Jointly Organised by The James Lind Alliance, The Social Science Research Unit, Institute of Education, University of London and the Royal College of Nursing Research Institute, University of Warwick, 20 November 2008. Available from: http://www.lindalliance.org/jla_ssru_rcni_outcomes_conference_nov_2008.asp. Accessed: 2 September 2010.
10. Valderas JM, Alonso J, Guyatt GH (2008) Measuring patient-reported outcomes: moving from clinical trials into clinical practice. *Medical Journal of Australia* **189**, 93–94.
11. Rimal RN, Lapinski MK (2009) Why health communication is important in public health. *Bulletin of the World Health Organization* **87**, 247.
12. Ajjawi R, Rees C (2008) Theories of communication. In: Higgs J, Ajjawi R, McAllister L, Trede F, Loftus S, (eds.) *Communicating in the Health Sciences.* Oxford University Press, South Melbourne, pp. 11–17.
13. McNab C (2009) What social media offers to health professionals and citizens. *Bulletin of the World Health Organization* **87**, 566.
14. Eccles MP, Armstrong D, Baker R, et al. (2009) An implementation research agenda. *Implementation Science* **4**, 18.
15. Lewin SA, Dick J, Pond P, et al. (2005) Cochrane Column, Commentary by G. Walt and RH. Morrow and author response. *International Journal of Epidemiology* **34**, 1250–1253.
16. Lewin S, Munabi-Babigumira S, Glenton C, et al. (2010) Lay health workers in primary and community healthcare for maternal and child health and the management of infectious diseases. *Cochrane Database of Systematic Reviews*, CD004015.
17. Lowe D, Ryan R, Santesso N, Hill S (In press) Development of a taxonomy of interventions to organise the evidence on consumers' medicines use. *Patient Education and Counseling*.doi:10.1016/j.pec.2010.09.024.
18. Weir M, Ryan R, Mayhew A, et al. The Rx for Change Database: a first-in-class tool for optimal prescribing and medicines use. *Implementation Science* **5**, 89.
19. Ryan R, Santesso N, Hill S, Lowe D, Kaufman C, Grimshaw J (2011) Consumer-oriented interventions for evidence-based prescribing and medicines use: an overview of systematic reviews. *Cochrane Database of Systematic Reviews*, CD007768.
20. Craig P, Dieppe P, Macintyre S, Mitchie S, Nazareth I, Petticrew M (2008) Developing and evaluating complex interventions: the new Medical Research Council guidance. *British Medical Journal* **337**, a1655.
21. Shepperd S, Lewin S, Straus S, et al. (2009) Can we systematically review studies that evaluate complex interventions? *Public Library of Science Medicine* **6**, e1000086.
22. Cochrane Consumers and Communication Review Group (2009) *Data Extraction Template for Cochrane Reviews.* Available from: http://www.latrobe.edu.au/chcp/assets/downloads/DET_2009update.doc. Accessed: 3 September 2010.

23. Ryan R, Prictor M, McLaughlin KJ, Hill S (2008) Audio-visual presentation of information for informed consent for participation in clinical trials. *Cochrane Database of Systematic Reviews,* CD003717.
24. Weston J, Hannah M, Downes J (1997) Evaluating the benefits of a patient information video during the informed consent process. *Patient Education and Counseling* **30**, 239–245.

CHAPTER 4

Identifying outcomes of importance to communication and participation

Sophie Hill[1], *Dianne B. Lowe*[2] *and Joanne E. McKenzie*[3]
[1]Coordinating Editor/Head, Cochrane Consumers and Communication Review Group, Centre for Health Communication and Participation, Australian Institute for Primary Care and Ageing, La Trobe University, Bundoora, Victoria, Australia
[2]Research Officer, Cochrane Consumers and Communication Review Group, Centre for Health Communication and Participation, Australian Institute for Primary Care and Ageing, La Trobe University, Bundoora, Victoria, Australia
[3]School of Public Health and Preventive Medicine, Monash University, Melbourne, Victoria, Australia

All health interventions are applied to people. This is self-evident, but it is not well recognised in the area of communication and participation that there are choices in how to communicate or involve people and some ways are better than others. It is critical to know what the consequences – outcomes – of an intervention are, because by implementing an intervention, an action or a strategy, we have intervened in someone's life [1]. Even the most benign-seeming communication intervention, an information pamphlet for instance, has an impact and may provoke anxiety in some readers and that anxiety may override the benefits of reading the information [2].

Chapter 2 heralded new roles for people regarding their health and its management. These roles indicate a breadth of social activity and relationships – as individuals, in families, as part of groups in the community and contributing to society's goals.

This breadth of roles and actions foreshadows the wide range of interventions or strategies for communicating with people and involving

The Knowledgeable Patient: Communication and Participation in Health – A Cochrane Handbook, First Edition. Edited by Sophie Hill.

them in all facets of decision-making about their health. These interventions were outlined in Chapter 3. Emphasis was given to clarifying the *purpose* of interventions for communication and participation. Being clear about the purpose is important because it sets the scene for finding out if what you intended to happen has actually happened [3].

This chapter looks at the types of outcomes we can expect from interventions to promote knowledgeable and involved consumers and carers. It looks at what outcomes have been measured in research and proposes a new taxonomy of outcomes of interventions for improving communication and participation. The taxonomy encompasses a comprehensive range and grouping of outcomes at consumer, provider and service levels. For example, it includes socially oriented outcomes, such as those related to communication and involvement, and clinically oriented or service outcomes, such as physical health or use of healthcare. This ensures that outcomes of importance to all parties are considered for analysis or future research.

Past research: what outcomes have been measured?

Health outcomes are defined as 'all the possible results that may stem from exposure to a causal factor, or from preventive or therapeutic interventions' [4]. Randomised controlled trials (RCTs) in healthcare typically examine the effect of an intervention (e.g. clinical treatments, medicines or procedures) on a set of outcomes for a group of participants with some condition. This is achieved by allocating participants by randomisation to a series of groups, often two, with each group of participants receiving a different intervention [5]. Outcomes measured may include those which were intended, but also unintended outcomes, such as harms. Important health outcomes would include mortality, morbidity, i.e. physiological or psychological health status, and quality of life. Outcomes may extend beyond the individual's health to include the use of services and resulting costs.

What are the types of outcomes of health communication and participation interventions that have been measured by RCTs in the past?

Traditionally, research in this field has tended to measure a small range of outcomes. Analysis of the Cochrane Consumers and Communication Review Group's register of over 3000 trials, specifically selected for their relevance to communication and participation, showed that health behaviour – in particular, patient compliance – was the most commonly measured outcome, and measured in more than one-third of the trials in the database. The two other most commonly measured outcomes were health status and well-being (in particular, psychological health), and knowledge and understanding (in particular, knowledge acquisition) (see Table 4.1).

Table 4.1 Past research: the top three outcomes measured in controlled trials of communication and participation interventions (no. of trials = 3623).

Outcome category	Most commonly measured outcomes	No. of trials in which outcome measured
Health behaviour	Compliance	1135
Reported in 2015 trials	Attitudes	654
	Health-enhancing lifestyle	391
	Use of intervention or services	348
	Risk-taking behaviour	283
Health status and well-being	Psychological health of the patient or carer	889
Reported in 1246 trials	Physical health of the patient or carer	314
	Psychosocial outcomes, e.g. quality of life	389
Knowledge and understanding	Knowledge acquisition	784
Reported in 873 trials	Retention of information	210
	Information access and use	18

Source: Cochrane Consumers and Communication Specialised Register of Controlled Trials; outcomes in 3623 trials coded. Trials may measure more than one outcome, September 2004.

Future research: a broader set of outcomes required

The outcomes of communication interventions may correspond to a wider range of health-related outcomes than has commonly been measured in RCTs in the past. The range of interventions outlined in Chapter 3 had a breadth of purposes: to inform, educate, communicate, support, skill, change behaviour, engage and seek participation of people in all spheres of health from individual to collective contexts. Recognising these diverse purposes leads to an argument for researchers, where appropriate, to select specific outcomes that come from a more comprehensive set of outcomes, including those which are relevant to consumers and carers.

It is also the case that interest in consumer empowerment has grown and new kinds of outcomes have emerged as outcomes which people want to achieve. For instance, clinicians, researchers and consumers have promoted and researched new ways of handling the medical encounter and discussing a prospective treatment with a patient so that the patient is an equal participant [6]. This has led to the concept of shared decision-making. Making a decision in a shared way is therefore a new type of outcome [7].

Consumers and carers have identified – and may value – different outcomes to those prioritised by health professionals [8–11]. This is the case for both physical and psychosocial functions [12] as it is for outcomes associated with communication interventions, for instance, people's information needs [13].

For these reasons, it is increasingly recognised that we need to consider a broader range of outcomes of interest to all healthcare decision-makers, including consumers, carers, healthcare professionals, organisations and policy makers [14]. In the longer term, this new direction will influence research as well as policy and service delivery.

A taxonomy of outcomes for communication and participation

In response to this need, the Cochrane Consumers and Communication Review Group developed an outcomes taxonomy [15] to provide a comprehensive (but not exhaustive) list of the main categories of outcomes relevant to communicating with and involving consumers in healthcare.

A taxonomy is a way of grouping like concepts or phenomena, organising them into groups or categories. It was developed from identifying the outcomes that had been measured in many controlled trials, and with discussion and feedback from editors with the Cochrane Consumers and Communication Review Group [16].

Main groups in the taxonomy

The outcomes taxonomy organises health outcomes into three main groups which are differentiated by their orientation (Table 4.2):

(a) consumer-oriented outcomes;
(b) healthcare provider-oriented outcomes; and
(c) health service delivery-oriented outcomes.

The word 'consumer' for group (a) does not refer just to one group of people in one type of role. Rather, it is used in the sense described in Chapter 2 – a conceptually and politically charged term to refer to people in various roles. In the context of an outcomes taxonomy of interventions for communication and participation, it could therefore refer to outcomes which have been measured in consumers occupying different roles, i.e. as members of the public, patients or family carers. Depending on the intervention, it could also include outcomes measured in people who are community volunteers or advocates. In other words, outcomes in the consumer group are outcomes which will be measured in patients, carers or members of the public, and similarly, outcomes in the healthcare provider group are those measured in health professionals, such as doctors, allied health therapists and nurses.

Table 4.2 Outcomes of importance to consumers, communication and participation: a new taxonomy.

Groups and orientation	Outcome category
(a) Consumer	Knowledge and understanding
	Communication
	Involvement in care
	Evaluation of care
	Support
	Skills acquisition
	Health status and well-being
	Health behaviour
	Treatment outcomes
(b) Healthcare provider	Knowledge and understanding
	Consultation processes
(c) Health service delivery	Service delivery level
	Related to research
	Societal or governmental

Groups and categories of outcomes

Table 4.2 sets out the main categories of outcomes for each of the three groups; i.e. each group is broken down into different categories of outcomes that are the result of various types of interventions for communication and participation:

(a) In the *consumer* group, there are nine broad outcome categories, spanning *knowledge* through to *treatment outcomes*.

The consumer group is the most detailed (compared with healthcare provider and health service delivery) because most of the interventions captured by the reviews coordinated by the Consumers and Communication Review Group are intending principally to change an aspect of a consumer's health. The taxonomy is built on the principle of placing consumers at the heart of communication and participation and so recognises that outcomes might encompass how people think, feel, act, interact or react. Outcomes of the social processes of communication and participation are therefore included along with health status outcomes.

(b) The *healthcare provider* group includes the categories of *knowledge and understanding* and *consultation processes* as the main categories of outcomes for health professionals from improving communication with and participation by consumers.

(c) The *health service delivery* group includes categories of outcomes at the *service delivery level*, those *related to research* and those at a *societal* or *governmental* level.

The outcomes in this group currently are very broadly framed. It is likely that more discrete outcome categories will emerge in this group in the future due to research into the outcomes of consumer participation in these arenas [17]. Outcomes at the societal level may be more difficult to quantify, but could still be an aim of interventions at individual or collective levels. For example, Osborne and colleagues argue that building people's capacity to self-manage their health and minimise the effects of disabling conditions may 'decrease "lost productivity"' or enhance the capacity of a community [18], although these outcomes are difficult to measure in a trial setting.

Types of outcomes in each category

In the taxonomy, each outcome category is broken down into more discrete types of outcomes, which are closer to the level at which the outcome will be measured. For instance, let us take the category *involvement in care* in the consumer group. Policies and interventions to improve the patient centredness of care often seek *involvement* or *patient* or *carer participation*. The outcome *involvement* may be a goal of many different types of interventions, such as case conferencing with patients and carers in a palliative care setting [19] or question checklists to help patients express their information needs in consultations [20]. Table 4.3 provides many of the types of involvement which have been measured in trials in the Consumers and Communication Group's database of trials.

Thinking about measuring outcomes

Each of the outcome categories and types may be broken down further in terms of how they are measured and in whom. Let us follow the path

Table 4.3 Types of consumer or carer involvement.

Group and orientation	Outcome category	Types of consumer or carer involvement measured in trials
(a) Consumer	Involvement in care	Decision-making process
		Decision support provided
		Decisions taken
		Decisional conflict
		Participant's perceptions of who made the decision(s)
		Satisfaction with the decisions made
		Clarity of values
		Agreement between personal values for outcome and choice
		Implementation of preferred choice
		Adherence to chosen option
		Patient and carer preferences
		Informed consent

Source: Cochrane Consumers and Communication Specialised Register of Controlled Trials, 2004.

of group: *Consumer* > Outcome category: *Involvement in care* > Outcome type: *Decisions taken.*

Examples of decisions at individual, service and community levels which consumers might have to take include the decision:

- to make healthy choices,
- to give informed consent,
- to share a decision,
- to seek care,
- to get vaccinated,
- to attend screening,
- to take a medicine,
- to refuse surgery,
- to volunteer to provide peer support,
- to participate in research and
- to make a complaint.

Depending on the intervention purpose and the type of decisions required, outcomes will be measured in different populations of people, e.g. old or young, healthy or sick, culturally diverse. They may be measured with people making different types of decisions, e.g. decisions for themselves or decisions on behalf of another, such as a parent making a decision for their young child.

Attributes of the trial population will therefore determine the type of measurement tool, or refinement of an existing tool, that is most appropriate for measuring that outcome. Measurement is a process whereby numbers are assigned 'to aspects of objects or events according to a rule of some kind' [21]. It is immediately obvious that this will create many challenges for people researching the effects of communication and participation. Can all that is meaningful about communication be reduced to a number? How can concepts such as trust [22], for instance, be turned into an outcome that can be measured in a way that produces findings that are valid (the measure reflects the concept it is intended to measure), reliable (the measure consistently produces the same results), as well as sensitive to degrees of change, and appropriate and acceptable in the study population [23]. It is not only the availability of valid measuring tools that creates challenges – there may be difficulties in interpreting this kind of outcome data; for instance, what is the meaning of a change, especially a small change?

In 2000, Bensing, a leading researcher in medical communication, wrote that the ideological basis of patient-centred medicine was better developed than its evidence base [24]. In a later conceptual paper with colleague de Haes [25], the researchers present a conceptual framework for outcomes, or endpoints as they term them, of interventions to improve medical communication. Serious challenges face those who want to build an evidence base from trials and systematic reviews about which interventions are effective. Challenges include the fact that many different health outcomes are being assessed and many different measurement scales are used to assess the same outcome. Many measurement scales do not have good measurement properties and there are outcomes which currently do not have measurement scales.

Given the many methodological and epistemological challenges, how can an outcomes taxonomy contribute to better research and, ultimately, better healthcare practice and improved health?

Using the taxonomy to identify outcomes of importance

The primary purpose of the taxonomy is to provide an overview of the range of outcomes relevant to the field of communication and participation, and to aid the process of thinking through the many different ways in which health for 'the knowledgeable patient' or 'the knowledgeable society' comes about (refer to Chapter 2).

The outcome categories are reflective of the range of interventions (see Chapter 3), including outcomes linked to interventions addressing personal autonomy and choice, interaction, social processes and capacities of both consumers and health professionals, health state outcomes, and service-related and societal effects.

Two main uses are identified:

1 *The taxonomy aids the identification of outcomes of importance to decision-makers:*

The taxonomy should aid the identification of outcomes of importance to decision-makers. This process is linked to how Cochrane reviews are conducted.

When conducting a Cochrane systematic review, authors must identify at the start of the research the main outcomes of the interventions of interest. The main outcomes are defined by the *Cochrane Handbook for Systematic Reviews of Interventions* as 'those that are essential for decision-making, and [which] should usually have an emphasis on patient-important outcomes' [26]. The choice of outcomes may be a decision based on theories of how the interventions work. It could be based on looking at past research. Increasingly, researchers are asking users of the intervention to identify important outcomes, and this could include policy makers, professionals, patients or carers [27]. Review authors then look to see if the trials included in their review have measured those specific outcomes. Pre-specifying outcomes at the start of a systematic review is done to minimise bias, since it reduces the risk of review authors selectively including the most 'favourable' results [28].

Decision-makers may place different degrees of importance on to different outcomes. Taking the example of self-management skills training to improve how people manage their medicines, the outcome of compliance is important to health professionals, but it figures less prominently in consumer research. A general practitioner (GP) may want to know if self-management skills help people take their medicines as directed (outcome = compliance, more recently termed 'adherence'). Consumers or carers, however, might want to know that training gives people the skills they need to manage various situations, such as knowing the purpose of the medicines, taking doses correctly and recognising side-effects, as well as taking medicines over time as prescribed (outcomes = knowledge, skills, minimising harms, compliance). Both parties will share an interest in the longer term health benefits of self-management strategies (outcome = health status and well-being). And new models of care which are socially and culturally informed, such as basing self-management education for asthma management in schools, may encourage researchers to measure social behaviour linked to illness or health (outcome = behaviour, i.e. school attendance) because this outcome will be of importance to teachers and parents [29].

The Cochrane Consumers and Communication Review Group promotes its outcomes taxonomy to authors to stimulate greater awareness of a broader range of outcomes than those that have been most commonly measured in the past. The group therefore uses the taxonomy as a tool to stimulate researchers to consider the range of outcomes which might be the result of the intervention and to consider the perspectives of different parties. In addition, Cochrane review authors are expected to identify any possible harms of the intervention and check the published papers of the trials to see if harms were reported. In this instance, the taxonomy may assist in identifying possible areas where harms may occur; e.g. *Evaluation of care* is a category that includes complaints as well as satisfaction. *Health status and well-being* is a category that includes anxiety as well as coping. It is hoped that consideration of the taxonomy by researchers will lead to inclusion of outcomes of importance to various parties.

2 *The taxonomy helps thinking through why (and how) complex interventions work:*

The second use is that the taxonomy may aid the process of thinking through how complex interventions work. In the past, researchers have concentrated largely on endpoint measures, such as cure or death. Measuring such outcomes is important, but it may tell you little about why an intervention has worked or not.

It is not always clear how complex social interventions, such as consumer or carer participation, have the effects they do. Street and colleagues trace pathways through which communication between the clinician and the patient can lead to improved health status [30]. Some pathways may be direct, for instance, the exchange of information in a consultation leads to the correct diagnosis, or some less direct, such as when an exchange of views leads to increased patient confidence to cope.

The Picker Institute Europe has been working with the NHS in England to identify the key domains of patients' experiences in hospitals [31]. The intention is to identify those aspects of people's experiences in acute care that have the strongest relationship to patients' overall satisfaction. Empirical research showed that most of the key domains and question areas which correlated with satisfaction revolved around the quality of people's interactions with doctors and nurses, the consistency of information provided, good coordination between doctors and nurses, receiving answers to questions that were understood, being involved in decisions and being treated with respect and dignity. The only domains which did not reflect different facets of communication were having pain controlled and the cleanliness of the hospital. This research provides a relationship between certain kinds of organised behaviour (e.g. coordination) and an outcome (e.g. satisfaction) and could underpin future research to test and compare whether different interventions to coordinate and communicate with patients lead to more or less satisfaction.

The taxonomy – in conjunction with theory – is useful for examining the mechanisms for why the intervention may or may not work. A complex intervention may have several facets or components. If it is effective, what is the mechanism of success, and does the entire package have to be implemented? How do we know if specific components work? Alternatively, if it does not work, do we know why and where the breakdown in effectiveness occurred? Would it be possible to modify one of the components?

Some of these questions are illustrated in the Cochrane review by Marteau and colleagues who examined the effects of communicating DNA-based disease risk. Does communicating DNA-based disease risk estimates lead to changes – in knowledge and understanding of risk status, to changes in perception of risk, in feelings of control with risk-reducing behaviour, of anxiety linked to fear of the disease, in intentions to change behaviour, in actual behaviour change (e.g. quitting smoking) and finally in longer term effects, such as a decrease in risk for heart disease [32]? If only the longer term outcomes are measured, and no change is apparent, do we know if people knew what to do and why, if people intended to change, or if they did change their behaviour, but it had no impact on their health.

A consistent language for outcomes of communication and participation

One other potential use for the taxonomy is to provide a consistent language to summarise the findings of systematic reviews for wider dissemination of information about evidence. For instance, the outcomes taxonomy could aid the summary presentation, dissemination and interpretation of effects from research on complex interventions. This is recognised as a key part of getting evidence into practice by making it more accessible and ensuring the most important messages are succinctly presented [33]. The Cochrane Consumers and Communication Review Group has used its outcomes taxonomy to summarise results from reviews for dissemination in evidence bulletins, accessible summaries of Cochrane reviews for decision-makers [34] (see Chapter 17). It has also used the taxonomy to create a consistent language for describing the effects of complex interventions, and this enables us to look across diseases, populations and settings. This has been done for the Canadian *Rx for Change* database of medicine-related review-level evidence, found at http://www.cadth.ca/index.php/en/compus/optimal-ther-resources/interventions.

Conclusion

As a conceptual framework, the Consumers and Communication Review Group's taxonomy is not used to make a judgement on the primacy or measurement properties of different outcomes or of the different ways of measuring outcomes. Regarding the latter, it does not differentiate between outcomes measured through objective means, such as measuring blood levels (following a medicine), and outcomes measured through subjective means, such as patients self-reporting how many medicines they have taken. This latter type of outcome is called a patient-reported outcome (or PRO) [35] and has been increasingly attracting attention [36], such as being allowed by the US Food and Drug Administration to support labelling claims for new medicines [37]. Objectively measured outcomes are considered in some situations to be more valid and reliable than outcomes reported by consumers [38]. However, the taxonomy's purpose is to signal many possible outcomes and not make a judgement about how those outcomes were measured or might be interpreted.

The key use of the outcomes taxonomy of the Cochrane Consumers and Communication Review Group is its function in supporting research. It therefore functions as a research tool, helping to build knowledge and flag knowledge gaps. It has the potential to be a resource for the production of new knowledge by being comprehensive in identifying outcomes associated with interventions for communication and participation.

References

1. Chalmers I (2003) Trying to do more good than harm in policy and practice: the role of rigorous, transparent, up-to-date evaluations. *The Annals of the American Academy of Political and Social Science* **589**, 22–40.
2. Hill S (2003) The Social Meanings of Being a Patient: A Sociological Analysis of the Experience of Surgery [PhD]. La Trobe University, Bundoora.

3. Nutbeam D (1998) Evaluating health promotion – progress, problems and solutions. *Health Promotion International* **13**, 27–44.
4. Last JM (ed.) (2001) *A Dictionary of Epidemiology*. Oxford University Press, Oxford.
5. Matthews JNS (2006) What is a randomized controlled trial. In: *Introduction to Randomized Controlled Clinical Trials*, 2nd ed. Chapman & Hall/CRC, Texts in Statistical Science.
6. Charles C, Gafni A, Whelan T (1997) Shared decision-making in the medical encounter: what does it mean? (Or it takes at least two to tango). *Social Science & Medicine* **44**, 681–692.
7. Duncan E, Best C, Hagen S (2010) Shared decision making interventions for people with mental health conditions. *Cochrane Database of Systematic Reviews*, CD007297.
8. Hill S (2003) What is new in health information? Evidence for health consumers and policy making. In: Lin V, Gibson B, (eds.) *Evidence-Based Health Policy: Problems and Possibilities*. Oxford University Press, South Melbourne, pp. 44–55.
9. Hill S, Stoelwinder J (2003) Communicating with consumers: the development of an evidence-based research agenda in chronic illness research. *Australian Journal of Primary Health* **9**, 218–222.
10. Goodare H (2006) The patient's perspective. *Health Expectations* **9**, 200–203.
11. Herbison P, Hay-Smith J, Paterson H, Ellis G, Wilson D (2009) Research priorities in urinary incontinence: results from citizens' juries. *BJOG: An International Journal of Obstetrics and Gynaecology* **116**, 713–718.
12. Hewlett SA (2003) Patients and clinicians have different perspectives on outcomes in arthritis. *The Journal of Rheumatology* **30**, 877–879.
13. Coulter A (1997) Partnerships with patients: the pros and cons of shared decision-making. *Journal of Health Services Research and Policy* **2**, 112–121.
14. PatientView (2008) *Outcomes in Clinical Research – Whose Responsibility?* Report of a seminar jointly organised by The James Lind Alliance, The Social Science Research Unit, Institute of Education, University of London and the Royal College of Nursing Research Institute, University of Warwick, 20 November 2008. Available from: http://www.lindalliance.org/jla_ssru_rcni_outcomes_conference_nov_2008.asp. Accessed: 2 September 2010.
15. Cochrane Consumers and Communication Review Group (2009) *Outcomes of Interest to the Cochrane Consumers and Communication Review Group*. Available from: www.latrobe.edu.au/chcp/assets/downloads/Outcomes.pdf. Accessed: 9 February 2010.
16. Stoelwinder J, Hill S, Oliver S, Broclain D, Wensing M, Brewer L (eds.) (2002) [P4] Coding Scheme for the Cochrane Consumers and Communication Review Group (CCCRG) Specialised Register. *10th Cochrane Colloquium*, 31 July – 3 August 2002. Available from: http://www.imbi.uni-freiburg.de/OJS/cca/index.php/cca/article/view/3688. Accessed: 20 December 2010.
17. Oliver SR, Rees RW, Clarke-Jones L, et al. (2008) A multidimensional conceptual framework for analysing public involvement in health services research. *Health Expectations* **11**, 72–84.
18. Osborne RH, Spinks JM, Wicks IP (2004) Patient education and self-management programs in arthritis. *Medical Journal of Australia* **180**, S23–S26.
19. Abernathy AP, Currow DC, Hunt R, et al. (2006) A pragmatic 2 × 2 factorial cluster randomized controlled trial of educational outreach visiting and case conferencing

in palliative care-methodology of the Palliative Care Trial [ISRCTN 81117481]. *Contemporary Clinical Trials* **27**, 83–100.

20. Kinnersley P, Edwards A, Hood K, et al. (2007) Interventions before consultations for helping patients address their information needs. *Cochrane Database of Systematic Reviews*, CD004565.
21. Cochrane Patient-Reported Outcomes Methods Group. Glossary. Available from: http://www.cochrane-pro-mg.org/Documents/CochraneGlossaryforuploadingtowebsiteFINAL.pdf. Accessed: 8 September 2010.
22. McKinstry B, Ashcroft R, Car J, Freeman GK, Sheikh A (2006) Interventions for improving patients' trust in doctors and groups of doctors. *Cochrane Database of Systematic Reviews*, CD004134.
23. Bowling A (2004) *Measuring Health: A Review of Quality of Life Measurement Scales*, 3rd ed. Open University Press, Berkshire.
24. Bensing J (2000) Bridging the gap. The separate worlds of evidence-based medicine and patient-centered medicine. *Patient Education and Counseling* **39**, 17–25.
25. de Haes H, Bensing J (2009) Endpoints in medical communication research, proposing a framework of functions and outcomes. *Patient Education and Counseling* **74**, 287–294.
26. Higgins J, Green S (eds.) (2009) Chapter 5. In: *Cochrane Handbook for Systematic Reviews of Interventions Version 5.0.2*. Available from: www.cochrane-handbook.org. Accessed: 14 April 2010.
27. Oliver S, Dezateux C, Kavanagh J, Lempert T, Stewart R (2004) Disclosing to parents newborn carrier status identified by routine blood spot screening. *Cochrane Database of Systematic Reviews*, CD003859.
28. Kirkham JJ, Altman DG, Williamson PR (2010) Bias due to changes in specified outcomes during the systematic review process. *Public Library of Science One* **5**, e9810.
29. Lassersson TJ, McDonald VM (2010) School-based self-management educational interventions for asthma in children and adolescents (Protocol). *Cochrane Database of Systematic Reviews*, CD008385.
30. Street R, Jr., Makoul G, Arora N, Epstein R (2009) How does communication heal? Pathways linking clinician-patient communication to health outcomes. *Patient Education and Counseling* **74**, 295–301.
31. Picker Institute Europe (2009) *Core Domains for Measuring Inpatients' Experience of Care*. Picker Institute Europe, Oxford.
32. Marteau TM, French DP, Griffin SJ, et al. (2010) Effects of communicating DNA-based disease risk estimates on risk-reducing behaviours. *Cochrane Database of Systematic Reviews*, CD14007275.
33. Lavis JN (2009) How can we support the use of systematic reviews in policymaking? *Public Library of Science Medicine* **6**, e1000141.
34. Ryan RE, Kaufman CA, Hill SJ (2009) Building blocks for meta-synthesis: data integration tables for summarising, mapping, and synthesising evidence on interventions for communicating with health consumers. *BMC Medical Research Methodology* **9**, 16.
35. Bowling A (2005) Measuring health outcomes from the patient's perspective. In: Bowling A, Ebrahim S, (eds.) *Handbook of Health Research methods: Investigation, Measurement and Analysis*. Open University Press, Berkshire, pp. 428–444.
36. Cella D, Riley W, Stone A, et al. (2010) The Patient-Reported Outcomes Measurement Information System (PROMIS) developed and tested its first wave of adult

self-reported health outcome item banks: 2005–2008. *Journal of Clinical Epidemiology* **63**, 1179–1194.

37. Speight J, Barendsee SM (2010) Editorial. FDA guidance on patient reported outcomes. *British Medical Journal* **340**, c2921.
38. Higgins J, Green S (eds.) (2009) Chapter 8. In: *Cochrane Handbook for Systematic Reviews of Interventions Version 5.0.2*. Available from: www.cochrane-handbook.org. Accessed: 14 April 2010.

CHAPTER 5
Communicating risk and risk statistics for preventing chronic disease

Sophie Hill[1], *Adrian G.K. Edwards*[2] *and Dianne B. Lowe*[3]
[1]Coordinating Editor/Head, Cochrane Consumers and Communication Review Group, Centre for Health Communication and Participation, Australian Institute for Primary Care and Ageing, La Trobe University, Bundoora, Victoria, Australia
[2]Professor in General Practice, Department of Primary Care and Public Health, School of Medicine, Cardiff University, Cardiff, Wales, United Kingdom
[3]Research Officer, Cochrane Consumers and Communication Review Group, Centre for Health Communication and Participation, Australian Institute for Primary Care and Ageing, La Trobe University, Bundoora, Victoria, Australia

Why was the research conducted?

Health communication is critical to preventing disease. Why is this so? Many chronic diseases are due to a combination of modifiable and non-modifiable risk factors. Examples of the former are smoking, poor diet, lack of exercise behaviour; examples of the latter are age, gender and genetics.

Health communication about risk has an equity dimension as well. This is because social and economic disadvantage is linked to poorer health. Disadvantage arises from the unequal distribution of the important social and economic determinants – income, employment, education, housing and environment – according to a World Health Organization report to the Commission on the Social Determinants of Health [1]. Precise causal relationships are not well understood.

Some have argued that socio-economic status (measured by education, income, occupation or other similar factors) is strongly associated with modifiable risk factors such as blood pressure, cholesterol, smoking and body mass index [2], which lead to increased mortality and morbidity. Socio-economic status is thought to influence mortality indirectly

The Knowledgeable Patient: Communication and Participation in Health – A Cochrane Handbook, First Edition.
Edited by Sophie Hill.

through behaviour and lifestyle determinants, environmental exposures through home and occupation, physical environments, and access to, use and quality of healthcare [3]. Limited education may result in less exposure to information about risk [4].

Strategies to reduce risk factors may be implemented at a population or societal level and also at an individual level. People cannot change risk factors unless they know about them, want to change them, understand how to change them and receive support and assistance in that process. This makes communication – and risk communication in particular – a key component of any strategy to reduce the impact of chronic disease, particularly where there are a number of known modifiable risk factors.

Cardiovascular disease (CVD) is a group of conditions and one of the main causes of mortality in the world, responsible for approximately 30% of total deaths in 2005 [5]. In Australian prevention guidelines, CVD refers to coronary heart disease, stroke and other vascular disease [6]. It is one of the top chronic disease prevention priorities for governments in the United Kingdom, Canada, USA, India, China and Australia [7].

Risk communication involves informing or educating people who are exposed to a risk factor (e.g. smoking) about their risk of disease. Information on the qualitative and quantitative dimensions of the risk may be presented with a view to enabling people to make decisions about changes in lifestyle or medications to reduce that risk [8]. A fundamental requirement for risk communication is to have concrete data from which to estimate the risk of an individual developing a disease. This is achieved by use of epidemiological research that has estimated the relationships between risk factors and the prevalence of a disease (the total number of cases at any one time). An example of a study that has been used to estimate the risk of a heart disease and stroke is the Framingham Heart Study [9] (see Box 5.1 for a brief history of the first and most influential longitudinal cohort study).

Risk communication is challenging for health professionals. General practitioners (GPs), and increasingly nurse practitioners, may be the first point of contact and information for many people. Apart from accurate calculation [10] and application to an individual patient, complex statistical concepts have to be communicated in ways that are easy to understand and motivating too [11]. Consumers' existing understandings of risk information, their individual personal life circumstances [12] and individual preferences for the formats used to communicate risk [13, 14] add another level of complexity.

This chapter presents findings from qualitative research into the views of health consumers and GPs on how risk for CVD should be discussed in consultations. The research was conducted as part of a larger project to explore preferences for different styles of risk communication ('representation') formats and was undertaken for the Australian Department of Health and Ageing [15]. Four focus groups were held with consumers

Box 5.1 The Framingham Heart Study

The Framingham Heart Study [5] is named after the town in Massachusetts, USA, where in 1948 a long-term cohort study was started (see www.framinghamheartstudy.org/). The Cochrane Collaboration's Glossary defines a cohort study as an observational study in which a defined group of people (the cohort) is followed over time. The outcomes of people in subsets of this cohort are compared to examine people who were exposed or not exposed (or exposed at different levels) to a particular intervention or other factor of interest (see www2.cochrane.org/resources/glossary.htm).

In Framingham, a large group of people – 5209 healthy men and women, aged 30 to 60 – were recruited to the study, undertook physical tests and interviews, and followed up every 2 years. Since then their children and grandchildren have joined the study. The risk factors for health disease and stroke were found to be high blood pressure, high blood cholesterol, smoking, obesity, diabetes and physical inactivity. These factors are universal, although varying in distribution across diverse populations.

Prior to the Framingham Heart Study, separate statistical models were used to calculate the risk of a specific CVD event for each risk factor separately. Looking at the effect of a single risk factor in isolation does not account for the interaction and multiplicity of these risk factors and how they ultimately affect people's health. Furthermore, such analyses focused on estimating an individual's likelihood of specific events over time, rather than their chances of developing *any* cardiovascular event, which may be more clinically important and more important in people's lives.

The Framingham Heart Study allowed for the analysis of multiple possible environmental and lifestyle factors to predict the risk of cardiovascular events over a 5- or 10-year time period using statistical models.

and four with GPs in both Melbourne metropolitan and rural areas in the state of Victoria. Consumers and GPs were asked similar questions. In this chapter, data from the consumer focus groups are used to examine what consumers say is important in risk communication. GPs' responses are used to examine the implications for health professionals.

What consumers said was important

In this section, the views of consumers from the focus groups are presented and discussed in the context of findings from research internationally. The topics follow a typical 'patient journey' from starting a conversation about risk to leaving the consultation and acting on the advice.

Starting the conversation about risk

Many of the participants were aware that risk factors would affect their general health. Information about cholesterol had been in the community long enough that some knew of the changing understanding of cholesterol, and recent debates about obesity had highlighted these issues more widely. No participant reported that their GP had used a CVD risk calculation tool with them, although many had their blood pressure and cholesterol tested and had been assessed for diabetes and one had undergone a bone density scan. Two people mentioned the benefits of having something concrete from a risk calculation tool, making the risk real.

Consumers' previous experiences of risk calculation:

> Because you [have] got a concise figure that you can work your way through ... for every centimetre you lose off your waist you decrease your risk of developing diabetes.
>
> §
>
> I had bone density scans for osteoporosis ... if you look at their graph it's really clear and it's actually a combination of those two [formats] ... it was a really good chart as I recall and what I can remember even now is ... where I fell on that chart ... so I could remember that ... because it was just visual.

The communication of risk information

Consumers unanimously expressed the view that risk information should be presented to them, even if knowledge could lead to shock. The level of detail varied though. People wanted clear explanations of what their risk factors were, why they were risk factors and how urgent/necessary the risk reduction action was. While some were trusting the GP's risk estimation, others wanted to know the evidence behind any suggestion that they were at risk. Despite research on shared decision-making emphasising the importance of disclosure of any uncertainties in the risk being communicated [16], no consumers raised this as an issue.

Consumers' responses to information about their risk of CVD:

> I think the GP has an obligation to tell you everything and some people may not be able to take that all in at once.
>
> §
>
> I'd be looking for a clear explanation of what the issue is.
>
> §
>
> I would take him at his word that he's a health professional, he knows a bit more about how the body operates than I do so I would have a

degree of trust in his expertise and I'd say to him, 'OK what is it exactly that I [have to] do?'

Some consumers commented on the changing evidence around modifiable risk factors. This has been identified as a potential barrier to patient action and an explanation for patients' inability to identify specific risk factors [17]. However, regular attention in the media to research findings and personal experience of changing views on the benefits of specific treatments meant that some were more aware of the source information behind the risk calculation tool. Perceived variation in research findings and the associated media coverage made it very difficult to determine which information could be trusted.

Consumer identification of CVD risk factors:

They're coming up with new ideas. There always seems to be a new thing out there that's being put out to us that it's the thing to do.

§

There's been far too much research and it's media hyping it all up or somebody promoting a book or whatever, so I've become very suspicious of research and data ... I want to know where this is all coming from.

Understanding the technical language and statistics of risk

Consumers were given risk formats that presented an absolute risk of a 55-year-old woman with a 16% risk of CVD in 5 years (i.e. absolute risk is the observed or calculated risk or rate of an event occurring in a defined population over a specified time period). This is a high-risk figure. Typically consumers had no existing reference point for the term 'absolute risk' and understood 'absolute' to mean 'complete'. They wanted it renamed to reflect a more personalised or individualised measure of risk.

Consumer understanding of the term 'absolute risk':

Personalised, I think that might hit home more than absolute. Absolute has strange connotations about what absolute could mean.

§

Or even verified, it's been verified, you have it like an experiment, a quantity of evidence that these things are a risk.

§

It makes sense but I don't like the absolute risk. Absolute risk – I can get in a car and I can get killed in a car and I might be in the right but someone could kill me. So that's absolute risk, isn't it?

Percentages were frequently misunderstood by consumers, hampering their understanding of the degree of risk. This is consistent with Gigerenzer's findings about the risks of misunderstanding with 'conditional probabilities', often because the 'reference class' – the group to which the risk refers – is not always clear [18]. Research indicates that it is more common for individuals to have difficulties with numeracy and find numbers more incomprehensible than not [19].

Participants did not readily grasp that 16% was high, and explanation and contextual cues such as age were important for comprehension. Health professionals' understanding of the size of risk would be quite different to consumers because of the training they have received.

Consumer preferences and (mis)understanding of presentation of risk formats:

> But that shows me that 20% is high and I wouldn't have thought that in the past.

Acting on the information: challenges for people in the 'real world'

Consumers with diabetes, who typically have a two- to fourfold increased risk of CVD, can both be unaware of and tend to overestimate their risk of future CVD [19]. As such, risk-reducing behaviours may not be adopted due to lack of awareness and overestimation of risk and may increase anxiety, which can hinder informed decision-making [19]. Although personalised risk estimation and risk factor identification itself may not lead to behaviour change, consumers in the focus groups acknowledged that this knowledge would be weighed up in the context of other factors. Previously identified barriers to behaviour change include complex personal social and economic factors [20], existing risk perceptions/misconceptions [12], optimism bias [21] and resistance to making many changes simultaneously.

There was recognition in the focus groups of the different responses GPs may encounter from patients, from scepticism to worry to acceptance. However, one theme emerging from several discussions was that the message given to patients needed to be clear and put strongly for them to believe it, but open ended enough to allow them to make choices and promote discussion about future action.

Consumer barriers or behaviour change in response to information about their risk of CVD:

> I think some people think they are invincible so they simply ignore it.
>
> §
>
> A lot of people, it seems to be that it has to get to a crisis before they will really do it [change their behaviour].
>
> §
>
> I would want it to be presented to me in a way that emphasised that I had a choice ... not just the heavy, 'if you don't do this you are going to die', but 'this is a very serious issue, you are not looking after your health but you've got choices in this' and ... 'these are the likely consequences'.

Communication extends beyond the consultation

People said they would like adequate information to take home following a discussion or calculation of CVD risk. Some also mentioned follow-up, with support to help them with possible shock or help them with recall of key information. However, this was not universally endorsed as a strategy, and for some, it was an added anxiety.

Consumers identified need for take-home CVD risk information:

> I was assuming ... that if this kind of tool were used that you would actually leave the doctor's surgery with little charts and graphs in your hands.
>
> §
>
> If the GP said 'I'll contact you' I think that would demonstrate a much greater concern and interest.
>
> §
>
> I don't know, I don't like reminders ... I've got to go to a spinal clinic every 12 months and I dread that every time it comes around.

The perspectives of GPs

This section presents the views of GPs in the focus groups and similarly follows the patient journey through the consultation. Relevant research from Ireland, the United Kingdom, Europe, USA and Australia informs the discussion.

Starting a risk communication discussion

Several GPs reported that in some circumstances it was very easy to talk with patients about CVD risk because community knowledge of risk issues was quite high. In other instances, GPs reported that it was difficult to discuss CVD risk and that it took time to broach the subject with particular patients. One way was to initiate a conversation about CVD risk from a discussion of blood pressure.

GPs on how to start a conversation about risk:

> Quite often people are quite keen to start talking ... because they've heard some of the story but they haven't actually taken it all on board and very often they are quite grateful actually to have the subject raised so they can have their questions answered.
>
> §
>
> I don't have any problem raising issues, but mainly they focus on cholesterol and that's more probably because we can do something about that. They're not really across the rest of the issues and that may be a form of denial in that [we will tell them] you've got to stop smoking, you've got to do it yourself, you are obese, you've got to do something about that

yourself, physical activity, you've got to do yourself, but blood pressure we can treat, so they're quite willing to do that.

The communication of risk information

GPs reported using a range of communication strategies in order to support a discussion about CVD risk with their patients. These methods were dependent on the individual, the presenting situation and the length of time they had known that patient.

Communication of risk information was favoured by some, rather than using risk calculation tools. For others, the main issues were to keep any discussion about CVD risk simple by using numbers sparingly, developing the relationship with the patient and checking how much the patient wanted to know. Experience varied as expected, with some patients seeking detailed information whilst others did not.

GPs mentioned that they would discuss factors such as smoking, blood pressure, dietary factors, cholesterol and non-changeable factors (age, gender and genetics) and what the patient could do about any risk factors they have, but not necessarily within the explicit context of CVD risk. Given this lack of context of risk discussions, it is not surprising that although consumers were reasonably knowledgeable about CVD risk factors, they did not always recognise them as risks associated specifically with CVD, but rather as more general health-related risk factors such as lack of exercise, cholesterol, smoking and stress. Despite 'stress' being a commonly used term, there is little consensus regarding the meaning of this term [22]; nonetheless, consumers in other studies have also perceived this to be a major risk factor for CVD [23].

GPs communicating risk factors:

> The most important thing is the interaction between you and the patient; the computer is a tool.
>
> §
>
> It can be really hard to pick what the motivational factors for each individual patient are going to be.

Communicating the technical language and statistics of risk

Clear visual representations of risk assists comprehension [19]. Consumers and GPs favoured the same four formats for risk information [15]. These included a statement, two vertical bar charts, one with more contextual information, and a line graph. Comparative and contextual cues were important for understanding the risk statistic. Having a range of formats available was important for GPs, who, like others in research, have stated they want some flexibility for discussion with different patients [24]. It also helps the doctor tailor risk information to the individual [13]. Whilst GPs' format preferences aligned with consumers, some felt that their patients did not respond well to numbers or charts. GPs also noted that if the information is personalised, the consumer takes notice of it. When discussing whether there were some formats that they would never use, several GPs said that they would never exclude any of the options, perhaps reflecting their experience and findings that any one risk communication format will not be unanimously preferred by all consumers [19, 25].

GP comments regarding using risk presentation formats:

> Well, we talk to patients in different ways depending on who they are and pick out the best ... once you're using a computer program you choose the level of sophistication appropriate to the patient ... If a racegoer came in you'd use [that option] ... the odds are.
>
> §
>
> I think you've got to be selective about these things. I think they can have a place but they have to be individualised and you have to choose your moment and if you've got different formats that are suitable for different people then they can be used selectively. But what I worry about with these things ... where you're trying to make a one size fits all ... [even with] the best of intentions it's hard [not to feel] ... that you were just trying to squeeze somebody into the same size.

Reflecting other research findings, and highlighting their own experiences of consumers' health literacy (or innumeracy), a number of GPs thought that the use of numbers, statistics, percentages, ratios and proportions was too difficult for some of their patients to understand or that their use might be confusing [25]. Several GPs also commented that since they did not understand particular numbers (such as odds) themselves, they would not expect that their patients would understand such measures accurately. Targeting particular groups may also be a strategy, recognising that some in the community were getting health information from other sources.

GP perceptions of consumer preferences and understanding:

> I think statistics leave most people cold .... People get used to statistics being twisted, it's politicians probably that make people very cynical of them and so I think in terms of figures, it just goes over people's heads.
>
> §
>
> I would not just say that to a patient, I would need to put it in a context ... now what does that mean to you?
>
> §
>
> One of the things we found in this ... study ... last year was that women are much better informed about health issues than men ... and I suspect that's because every women's magazine now has a health page.

Behaviour change: challenges for people in the 'real world'

GPs in the focus groups identified that they used various strategies to take account of the patient's educational level, patient circumstances and culture, and opportunities to raise risk. While some individuals possess a good understanding of risk factors, they also show little motivation to change their behaviour [26]. This may reflect ambivalence to the methods and goals of risk reduction, described as relating to five different stages of perceiving risk and adopting behaviour change strategies (perception, demand, information, priority and treatment ambivalence) [27]. Yet, within the focus groups, several consumers had already taken action to reduce risk, even though they could not recall receiving an explicit previous message about their own CVD risk.

GPs used many different techniques to motivate their patients to change their behaviour, including discussing the patient's family history of CVD, using fear messages, visual aids, focusing on a patient's achievements and other patient successes, talking about future quality of life, and following up with patients.

Indicating a level of frustration with the size and responsibility of their task, many GPs suggested that public health community education campaigns may help to relieve their responsibility to educate, motivate and sustain the wider community about health-related matters, including CVD risk.

GP identified issues regarding patient motivation and behaviour change:

> I think the other thing with motivational behaviour is it varies over time. I've been in a practice for well over 20 years so I've seen people over that time who are in risk and their risk factors have gone up and down due to the way they are at that point in time.
>
> §
>
> I often try and look at other things in their life that would be motivating factors for them.

Communication extends beyond the consultation

GPs reported that take-home information (particularly dietary information) is given to patients, to help recall and encourage them to return to ask any further questions. However, not all patients wanted to be followed up, so gaining patient consent for this process was necessary.

GPs identified need for take-home information:

> Usually we get them [information sheets] from our computer ... and give them the information. There are lots of brochures about diet, cholesterol ... which are very useful I think.

Conclusion

This chapter has plotted the different ways in which risk communication can be raised and discussed in a GP consultation, with the themes tying in with national priorities to ensure that preventive opportunities are not missed [28]. Data were presented which follow a typical journey – from starting a conversation and communicating risk to dealing with the challenges of how to aid understanding, provide support for acting on the information and for communication beyond the consultation.

Risk communication is important. It is one way of raising consumers' perceptions of the importance of risk factors and their ability to modify at least some of these. A range of ways of communicating risk is probably necessary to account for individual variation in perception and understanding [15]. Supporting the conversation about risk and risk reduction options will enable consumers to decide on specific strategies to reduce risk, enabling the focus to move on to implementation (and maintenance) of behaviour change.

References

1. Kelly MP, Morgan A, Bonnefoy J, Butt J, Bergman V (2007) *The Social Determinants of Health: Developing an Evidence Base for Political Action*. Final Report to the World Health Organization Commission on the Social Determinants of Health, Universidad del Desarrollo, Chile and National Institute for Health and Clinical Excellence, United Kingdom. Available from: http://www.who.int/social_determinants/resources/mekn_final_report_102007.pdf. Accessed: 25 August 2010.
2. Winkleby MA, Cubbin C, Ahn DK, Kraemer HC (1999) Pathways by which SES and ethnicity influence cardiovascular disease risk factors. *Annals of the New York Academy of Sciences* **896**, 191–209.
3. Reiner AP, Carlson CS, Ziv E, Iribarren C, Jaquish CE, Nickerson DA (2007) Genetic ancestry, population sub-structure, and cardiovascular disease-related traits among African-American participants in the CARDIA Study. *Human Genetics* **121**, 565–575.
4. Adler NE, Newman K (2002) Socioeconomic disparities in health: pathways and policies. *Health Affairs* **21**, 60–76.
5. Commission on Social Determinants of Health (2008) Closing the Gap in a Generation: Health Equity Through Action on the Social Determinants of Health. *Final Report of the Commission on Social Determinants of Health,* World Health Organization, Geneva.
6. National Vascular Disease Prevention Alliance (2009) *Guidelines for the Assessment of Absolute Cardiovascular Disease Risk.* National Heart Foundation of Australia. Available from: http://www.heartfoundation.org.au/SiteCollectionDocuments/A_AR_Guidelines_FINAL%20FOR%20WEB.pdf. Accessed: 26 October 2010.
7. Global Alliance for Chronic Disease (2009) *Fact Sheet on Global Alliance for Chronic Diseases.* Available from: http://www.ga-cd.org/. Accessed: 26 October 2010.
8. Risk Communication (2007) *A Dictionary of Public Health.* Oxford University Press. Available from: http://0-www.oxfordreference.com.alpha2.latrobe.edu.au/

views/ENTRY.html?subview=Main&entry=t235.e3949. Accessed: 11 January 2010.

9. Dawber TR, Meadors GF, Moore FE, Jr. (1951) Epidemiological approaches to heart disease: the Framingham Study. *American Journal of Public Health* **41**, 279–281.
10. Torley D, Zwar N, Comino EJ, Harris M (2005) GPs' views of absolute cardiovascular risk and its role in primary prevention. *Australian Family Physician* **34**, 503–504, 507.
11. van Steenkiste B, Van Der Weijden T, Stoffers HE, Kester AD, Timmermans DR, Grol R (2007) Improving cardiovascular risk management: a randomized, controlled trial on the effect of a decision support tool for patients and physicians. *European Journal of Cardiovascular Prevention and Rehabilitation* **14**, 44–50.
12. Grol R, Grimshaw J (2003) From best evidence to best practice: effective implementation of change in patients' care. *Lancet* **362**, 1225–1230.
13. Edwards A, Elwyn G, Gwyn R (1999) General practice registrar responses to the use of different risk communication tools in simulated consultations: a focus group study. *British Medical Journal* **319**, 749–752.
14. Edwards A, Elwyn G, Wood F, Atwell C, Prior L, Houston H (2005) Shared decision making and risk communication in practice: a qualitative study of GPs' experiences. *The British Journal of General Practice* **55**, 6–13.
15. Hill S, Spink J, Cadilhac D, et al. (2010) Absolute risk representation in cardiovascular disease prevention: comprehension and preferences of health care consumers and general practitioners involved in a focus group study. *BMC Public Health* **10**, 108.
16. Elwyn G, Edwards A, Kinnersley P, Grol R (2000) Shared decision making and the concept of equipoise: the competences of involving patients in healthcare choices. *British Journal of General Practice* **50**, 1923–1932.
17. Gigerenzer G, Gaissmaier W, Kurz-Milcke E, Schwartz L, Woloshin S (2008) Helping doctors and patients make sense of health statistics. *Psychological Science in the Public Interest* **8**, 53–96.
18. Gigerenzer G, Edwards A (2003) Simple tools for understanding risks: from innumeracy to insight. *British Medical Journal* **327**, 741–744.
19. Price HC, Dudley C, Barrow B, Kennedy I, Griffin SJ, Holman RR (2009) Use of focus groups to develop methods to communicate cardiovascular disease risk and potential for risk reduction to people with type 2 diabetes. *Family Practice* **26**, 351–358.
20. Facione NC, Dodd MJ, Holzemer W, Meleis AI (1997) Helpseeking for self-discovered breast symptoms. Implications for early detection. *Cancer Practice* **5**, 220–227.
21. Price PC, Pentecost HC, Voth RD (2002) Perceived event frequency and the optimistic bias: evidence for a two-process model of personal risk judgments. *Journal of Experimental Social Psychology* **38**, 242–252.
22. Bunker SJ, Colquhoun DM, Esler MD, *et al.* (2003) 'Stress' and coronary heart disease: psychosocial risk factors. *The Medical Journal of Australia* **178**, 272–276.
23. Farooqi A, Nagra D, Edgar T, Khunti K (2000) Attitudes to lifestyle risk factors for coronary heart disease amongst South Asians in Leicester: a focus group study. *Family Practice* **17**, 293–297.
24. Edwards A, Matthews E, Pill R, Bloor M (1998) Communication about risk: diversity among primary care professionals. *Family Practice* **15**, 296–300.

25. Edwards A, Matthews E, Pill R, Bloor M (1998) Communication about risk: the responses of primary care professionals to standardizing the 'language of risk' and communication tools. *Family Practice* **15**, 301–307.
26. Gabhainn SN, Kelleher CC, Naughton AM, Carter F, Flanagan M, McGrath MJ (1999) Socio-demographic variations in perspectives on cardiovascular disease and associated risk factors. *Health Education Research* **14**, 619–628.
27. Kehler D, Christensen B, Lauritzen T, Christensen MB, Edwards A, Risor MB (2008) Ambivalence related to potential lifestyle changes following preventive cardiovascular consultations in general practice: a qualitative study. *BMC Family Practice* **9**, 50.
28. Kehler D, Christensen B, Lauritzen T, Christensen MB, Edwards A, Bech Risor M (2008) Cardiovascular-risk patients' experienced benefits and unfulfilled expectations from preventive consultations: a qualitative study. *Quality in Primary Care* **16**, 315–325.

CHAPTER 6

What does participation mean? Reshaping our understanding of the meaning of surgery

Sophie Hill[1] *and Jessica Kaufman*[2]

[1]Coordinating Editor/Head, Cochrane Consumers and Communication Review Group, Centre for Health Communication and Participation, Australian Institute for Primary Care and Ageing, La Trobe University, Bundoora, Victoria, Australia

[2]Research Officer, Cochrane Consumers and Communication Review Group, Centre for Health Communication and Participation, Australian Institute for Primary Care and Ageing, La Trobe University, Bundoora, Victoria, Australia

Why was the research conducted?

To be a patient is to participate in one of society's major social institutions: health services. This chapter examines the social meanings of being a patient in a modern society by analysing patients' views of their experiences of undergoing treatment. This information was gathered through interviews with 30 people who underwent a serious surgical procedure in order to treat carotid stenosis, a narrowing of the carotid artery that supplies blood to the brain. We focus on surgical patients' views of the entire experience, their actions and decisions, their communication with doctors and the process of treatment.

Despite the wealth of research related to health participation, there are far less studies in which people are asked how they feel about having the illness or treatment. Why do researchers baulk at immersing themselves in the 'social world' of their patients? We might learn something from listening to people's voices.

The research included in this chapter is drawn from a thesis written by Hill in 2003 [1]. Jessica Kaufman has explored the implications for

The Knowledgeable Patient: Communication and Participation in Health – A Cochrane Handbook, First Edition. Edited by Sophie Hill.

shared decision-making. The research examines the nature and meanings of the experience of surgery qualitatively through in-depth interviews with people aged 53 to 93, living in Melbourne or rural Victoria, Australia. Ethics approval was granted by the ethics committees of the university and the two hospitals involved in the study. The names of all participants were changed to ensure confidentiality.

Participation contexts and styles and preferences for information are now discussed, followed by implications for health professionals. The chapter concludes with a summary of the sociological concepts generated by the qualitative analysis. By analysing the interview data, three overarching patterns were identified, characterised by varying attitudes towards health assessment, medical treatment and healthcare professionals.

Participation in surgical and medical treatment for carotid stenosis

Consumer participation occurs whenever an individual engages with the health system. The most recognised form of patient participation may be the doctor–patient exchange which occurs during a consultation, but there are other contexts in which participation occurs and is often overlooked.

In this chapter, consumer participation is examined from the patient's perspective. From these first-person experiences, we can identify contexts, styles, needs and preferences for participation and information exchange.

Contexts for participation

Symptom assessment

Dealing with illness can carry a person through many stages of participation. The individuals quoted in this chapter all had variations of the same condition, but their interaction with the health system began in different ways.

Most people experienced one or more symptoms of what would be determined to be a narrowing of the carotid artery. Some assessed their symptoms and sought medical attention immediately. These people were *ready* to act, and may have even *initiated* action. The way they described their experiences and views indicated their readiness and, in some cases, their preference for swift medical action:

> I was going for me walks with the dog next door and me legs, after about 500 yards, me legs got a bit funny and discomfort, no hard pains . . . I was getting them about three times a day. And I said, 'There's something wrong here, this is angina I reckon' and went to me local GP. (Mr. Borg)

Others were more *uncertain* and hesitant to take this first step towards interaction, and although they experienced symptoms, they did not immediately recognise them to be cause for concern. One woman describes an experience in which she fell over after her right leg went numb:

> At this stage, I didn't understand the significance of it at all ... and I thought oh, I'll just sit here for a minute and I won't bother him [her husband] at all and I'll get up on my merry way but of course it didn't come good. (Mrs. Sherbrook)

She went to the hospital, but was still reluctant to accept the seriousness of her condition. She said to the doctor:

> 'Couldn't I just stay at the farm for the weekend and I'll come back on Monday' and he said, 'That's the most appalling thing that I've ever heard.' (Mrs. Sherbrook)

Although the timeframe for initial participation varied significantly, most people sought medical treatment after experiencing symptoms. However, some individuals never experienced any symptoms at all, and their participation began in a different way. These individuals were diagnosed by doctors during examinations, with the news sometimes coming as a surprise. The subsequent participation of these asymptomatic people was often characterised by an increased willingness to be guided by the recommendation of the doctors.

> [The doctors] seemed quite amazed really that there were no symptoms, you know, but there was nothing there out of the ordinary, as far as I was concerned .... So they thought, at the time, or [the neurologist] thought at the time, that it was the time to have it done and of course he sent me back to [the surgeon] and [he] said the same thing. So we went and had it done. (Mr. Harris)

Decision-making

Regardless of how they assessed or did not assess their symptoms, all the patients interviewed were eventually faced with decisions regarding surgery and medical treatment. Carotid endarterectomy surgery involves opening the patient's neck and carotid artery to remove plaque from the arterial wall. It may be performed under local or general anaesthesia, and carries serious risks, including stroke, death, nerve damage and bleeding. People had to decide when to seek medical attention and advice, whether to have surgery and whether that surgery would be with local or general anaesthesia. Patterns of action similar to those found in symptom assessment emerged in the way in which they approached the decision-making process.

One group of people experienced a rapid transition from symptom recognition to surgery patient. They discussed their fears and how frightened they were, but there was no discussion of resistance or ambivalence, uncertainty or regret. Their relationships with their clinicians were characterised by a shared sense of task or responsibility, which was made evident by their almost seamless transitions from noticing the first symptom to being admitted for surgery.

> When they told me, you need an operation, I said okay, when? Monday! Okay, I said no worries, about it . . . . (Mr. Katakis)

For others, there was a sense of uncertainty about the experience. There was no sense of decision-making moving in tandem with doctors or nurses, as with the first group. Participants expressed their ambivalence about agreeing to have surgery, using phrases such as 'I sort of, I know I had to be sensible', 'I guess a good decision in the end', 'Perhaps I was fairly fortunate' and 'I thought I'd go along with it'. In contrast to members of the first group, they did not assert the need for action inherent in the phrase, 'Let's get it done'.

Surgery

The participation of the patient in surgery is often overlooked by researchers and health professionals, but for the seven people who had local anaesthesia and were awake during their procedures, the experience was significant. It was profound in itself and it also contributed to their overall understanding of their illness and treatment. They did not need the surgery interpreted for them by the doctor retrospectively – they *knew* what the operation was like, rather than having woken from an experience that had happened *to* them. There was a complete intersection with the procedure of surgery.

This experience was reasonable or bearable for most, giving some a sense of participating in the actual treatment. It meant that they were awake and monitoring how their body was opened. It was an experience that required courage, particularly given the lack of prior experience. One woman found it empowering and one man said he got bored. The memories of the time could be very visceral as well as confronting because patients could hear the actual process of being cut open, they could hear the surgical team talking (or hear the silence) and they had to respond to questions so that their progress could be monitored.

In a few cases, the patients were uncomfortable about something during the surgery and wanted to speak up, but felt that there was not an opportunity to do so. One man describes an experience he found 'humiliating', in which he urinated during the operation:

> You don't want to interrupt because there's a fair bit of attention. *[Yes.]* . . . I would have liked to interrupt them about the urine business but . . . it's a bit sort of humiliating, isn't it? (Mr. Cummins)

People's assessments of the actual process of surgery could provide doctors with additional information to guide practice. For example, patients may experience anxiety due to unusual sounds or even silences in the operating theatre, as well as the content of conversations overheard between doctors.

Where there was a choice about form of anaesthesia, and participants chose the general, one major reason was that they did not feel that they could be awake if something bad happened.

> How would I have been like, you know, with that local anaesthetic down there and they've suddenly walked in and gone, 'Oh Christ! This is a lot worse than it was!' I would have been on the floor. (Mr. Prentice)

This experience would have been too overwhelming. They did not wish, therefore, to intersect with the actual process of surgery.

After surgery

So much of the attention of the patient and the doctor is focused on the period up to and including surgery that there is little emphasis placed on postoperative participation. The time after surgery can be troubling, particularly if people experience adverse side effects or if new symptoms arise. One man developed pain around his eyes after the procedure, but his doctor's explanation of its cause left him uncertain and confused.

> 'I've got pain there', and he said, 'Tension'. Everybody told me tension. What tension! I don't have tension. (Mr. Katakis)

Several people who had faced surgery with confidence and readiness became more uncertain afterwards. Even though they had survived a dangerous experience, they were more aware of the possibility of future risk and ill health, particularly if they developed new symptoms or other illnesses. A man who had suffered a small stroke during surgery struggled to come to terms with the fact that he had experienced the rare possible side effect he had been warned about:

> I can't believe I fell into the 2% chance of having a stroke . . . . (Mr. Denver)

Others who had been very frightened before the procedure were able, upon its successful completion, to make sense of the experience. After surgery, one woman immediately read the information pamphlet that had been provided to her before the operation, but which she had been too nervous to read earlier.

Participation styles

The different *contexts* or *stages* of the illness experience – *when* participation occurs – are described above. This section explores the different *styles* of patient participation identified in the analysis – i.e. *how* participation occurs.

Initiation

This is the most active form of participation. Patients who *initiate* participation assert the existence of symptoms, start a discussion in favour of a specific course of treatment and ask questions assertively.

> I try to get as much out of them as I can without being cheeky, but I ask questions and expect an answer. (Mr. Rue)

Linked to this kind of independent action is the notion of independent relations with doctors. This may lead to challenging behaviour. The patient is not in awe of medical authority, and may be sufficiently confident to challenge medical opinion.

> Well I just said I wanted it [the operation]. [Right.] I said. 'No', he said, 'You don't want it' and I said, 'I believe I do'. (Mr. Rodwell)

Silence is not a characteristic of this form of participation.

Agreement

This participation style is characterised by a readiness to act. The language of *agreeing* is straightforward: 'It must be done', 'Let's get it done', 'Run with it'.

Active agreement implies an individual informed according to need. This means that patients feel comfortable interacting with doctors, but may also choose to be silent.

> I was given as much information as I wanted, no more, no less. And that suited me down to the ground. (Mr. Denver)

Neither medical authority is experienced as oppressive, nor is it challenged. Instead, patients have a sense of their equal worth. Ease of relations is reflected in the preferred communication styles of doctors: straightforward, informative but not exhaustively so, and non-judgemental.

> He's a man you can talk to and he'll answer questions .... Won't try and dodge them. (Mr. Rumble)

Acceptance

Patients whose participation is characterised by a sense of uncertainty can be described as *accepting* the need to act, rather than initiate or agree with action.

This form of participation may entail considerable strain. There may be resistance to the newly acquired information of risk, reluctance to ask questions or raise concerns, and dissatisfaction with the communication styles of doctors or information provided. This resistance is not total, however. Choice and acceptance of treatment is still made, but it may be a reluctant choice, or the strain of the overall experience may remain after its completion. The strain of the experience may mean that people readily complain about aspects of their treatment, such as the rudeness of students, costs of treatment or threatening way information is provided.

> [The doctor and medical students] sort of spoke about me as third person and oh, very embarrassing actually and I didn't like to interrupt, I didn't like to say anything because here he is explaining to his students, and didn't ask him any questions, so I didn't. (Mrs. Waverley)

Medical authority may be seen as oppressive, and there is no sense of shared task or decision-making moving in tandem. Fear may engender silence, making it more difficult to ask for desired information (see Chapter 1).

> I never seem to have the right questions because when I come home I always got plenty that I should have – I believe I should have asked. (Mr. Rodwell)

Fear may also mean that the information provided is insufficient or cannot be taken in when it is provided.

Information preferences

A key feature of health participation and decision-making is informing people according to need. This includes tailoring to the audience by varying the quantity, timing and format of information to suit the preferences of individuals [2, 3].

Family

Several people involved their family members in the information exchange process. Some were too frightened to read information pamphlets and instead passed them along to family members. For one man, the involvement of his family was suggested by his surgeon. The man's satisfaction with the surgeon was boosted by the surgeon's willingness to explain the operation to the man's family.

> [The surgeon], prior to the operation, he said, 'If your family want to know about, all about', he said, 'we'll make an appointment, get together', and said, 'I'll explain the lot to them'. He explained the whole operation, the whole procedure ... I knew I had a good surgeon, and had the confidence there. (Mr. Derbyshire)

Amount of information

People had very different preferences in regard to the amount of information they wanted from their doctors. Some people who wanted a great deal of detailed information found it difficult to obtain, but most were informed to a degree that they found satisfactory.

Contrary to what might be expected, patients who met with several different specialists or other clinicians could find it difficult to get enough information from any of them.

> Well, I wanted to ask the [technician] who was doing the carotid but he said, 'It'll be explained to you by the next person', but they didn't explain anything and I couldn't find out anything. (Mr. Missen)

For people who did not necessarily want to know everything that was going to happen, their doctor's intention to inform them was still important.

> Dr – was straightforward and treated me [as] a person with a little bit of intellect, anyhow and I didn't ask him anything about it and he said, 'Do you want to know anything about it?' and I said 'No'. (Mr. Haywood)

Timing

Several people expressed a strong preference to receive information at the end of their experience, after surgery rather than before it. Before the procedure, the information was too frightening to read, but learning about it later helped them make sense of the experience.

> Then after, when I could think about it, I was very glad to read all that. [In the pamphlet?] Yes. I thought it was very good. It more or less tells you everything you want to know. (Mrs. Brooks)

Some other patients sought as much information as possible before the operation, even performing their own research to add to that which was provided by their physicians.

Information-seeking behaviour and the type of information needed by an individual can also change over time with the addition of multiple new diagnoses. The accumulation of illness could mean that a person became too sick and tired to look for or process detailed information. Mrs. Nicoll, for example, underwent three major surgical operations in 3 months. Before the first surgery, a triple bypass, she was very informed.

> I was sort of prepared. I'd read everything. Everything I could get to read, I read about it. (Mrs. Nicoll)

By the time she underwent the carotid endarterectomy, however, she had a very different attitude regarding the level of information she required.

> I didn't know anything .... I think I buried my head in the sand and I take everything as it comes. (Mrs. Nicoll)

Format

Not all the patients preferred to receive information from their doctors exclusively. Two men wanted to speak to patients who had undergone the same surgery earlier to supplement the figures and percentages provided by the doctors.

> There was a chap in there, I see the scar on his left side. I started asking him about it. He give me confidence and one of the nurses at the private hospital told me her father had one done with no complications and that kept building me confidence up. (Mr. Borg)

Another man looked to medical books on his own to work out what was happening. He felt it was important to take responsibility, not only for his health but also for what he could find out. He used his knowledge and self-awareness of his health to initiate tests and treatment.

> I'd say, if I want to learn anything, I'll read a book and I think that's the way you find out ... you can't always take the word of anyone. (Mr. Prentice)

Implications of the findings for health professionals

Shared decision-making

Shared decision-making is a model of the physician–patient relationship in which both parties have an equal role in determining the course of treatment. Although the literature supplies varying definitions for shared decision-making [4–6], the model put forth by Charles and colleagues is widely cited as the foundational definition for the concept [4]. According to Charles, shared decision-making is characterised by four features: it involves at least the patient and the physician (though additional people may join the process); both parties share information, contribute to the treatment decision and agree upon the final treatment choice. Makoul's systematic review of shared decision-making definitions led to an integrated definition including some additional elements, particularly that the discussion of the patient's willingness and ability to follow a given course of action is also critical in determining the most appropriate option [5].

This concept informs many areas of clinical practice, including the development of decision aids, forms of risk communication, new health policies and training for clinicians [6]. Acute care decisions, such as those related to urgent surgery as described above, are sometimes seen as situations in which shared decision-making is not applicable [7]. Decisions must be made very quickly, and often there is no treatment choice, except whether or not to have the procedure.

The research showed that despite the unique decision-making circumstances of surgery, elements of shared decision-making are still relevant and valuable. For instance, information such as treatment options and consequences, patient values and relevant history must be shared between both the physician and the patient, and patients still participate in the treatment decision process and agree to the final decision. People valued the opportunity to ask questions to their doctors, and were frustrated when they could not get answers or when they were not given the chance to ask. The people who expressed high levels of satisfaction with their experiences were those who felt that their physicians treated them as equals and that their treatment decision was made with input from both the physician and the patient. Positive health outcomes, including symptom resolution and pain control, have been linked to effective communication and agreement between the physician and the patient [8,9]. Decision aids and other participation tools are most effective when combined with collaborative doctor–patient interaction [2]. Health professionals should be given the resources and training necessary to improve and develop their communication skills and enable them to encourage a shared decision-making approach in patient consultations [10].

Awareness of people's participation in surgery itself

The research described in this chapter identified the conscious experience of surgery as an underrecognised context for patient participation. Patients commonly experience fear, anxiety and discomfort relating to surgery and anaesthesia [11]. The primary context for addressing these concerns and delivering information to the patient is during the pre-operative visit [12]. When the procedure is performed under general anaesthesia or with sedation, the next participation interaction occurs during the postoperative consultation. For patients undergoing surgery with local anaesthesia, however, the surgery itself becomes an intermediate context in which they participate. The heightened emotions and physical vulnerability of surgery along with the unfamiliar environment of the operating theatre can make this participation experience very intense, as shown here and by Mauleon and colleagues, who researched the experience of hip surgery [11].

Searches reveal very few studies regarding patient experience or participation in surgery with local anaesthesia. First-hand interview information is the primary source of information highlighting areas of concern and ways to improve the surgery participation process. It is important for clinicians to recognise that patients under local anaesthesia are experiencing a range of sensations and emotions, and these may vary significantly based on the demographics and participation styles of the individuals undergoing surgery, as well as the length and nature of the procedure itself [1,12].

Communication and lack of communication can affect a patient's experience, whether it is between the patient and the physician or amongst physicians [8]. Several of the carotid endarterectomy patients found it difficult to speak up about their concerns during the operation. A woman was frightened when she heard the surgeons discussing another patient who had been diagnosed with cancer. Several other patients indicated that periods of silence could be stressful because they did not know what was going on around them. These issues indicate that clinicians may see surgery as a non-interactive environment, and they may neglect to attend to the patient's participation needs as they would in consultations. One way to address this is to have a dedicated person to talk to the patient throughout the surgery; 92% of respondents in a study in which this concept was tested found it reassuring [13].

The unfamiliar setting and sensations of the operating theatre may also disturb some patients. A study conducted by Mauleon and colleagues [11] featured interviews with older patients who underwent hip replacement or repair procedures with local anaesthesia. The study identified a theme of 'compromised well-being and comfort' experienced by the patients during surgery. This theme was characterised by pain, a sense of endless waiting and time dilation, a feeling of unreality and varying feelings of trust and distrust. Some carotid endarterectomy patients used words such as 'tense' or 'boring' to describe how they felt during the operation. One felt claustrophobic under the anaesthesiologist's curtain.

Several people had strong memories of the physical aspects of the surgery, such as hearing skin tear and feeling surgeons 'sucking the blood out'. Clinicians should be conscious of the fact that patients may feel things they are not prepared for and may need reassurance or explanation during surgery in order to address these sensations.

Despite their concerns and anxieties, the patients who underwent the surgery with local anaesthesia were satisfied with their decision. Their overall assessment of the experience varied from tolerable to good. This reflects the findings of a study of 1000 carotid endarterectomy surgeries with local anaesthesia, in which 91% of respondents said they had no problems with the experience and 93% would choose local anaesthesia again for similar surgery [14].

Timing of information delivery

Information regarding surgery is typically delivered in one or more preoperative consultations, in the form of patient–physician discussion and sometimes written or audio-visual materials [2, 8, 15].

Some people find that they can process information only after they have gone through surgery and are no longer dealing with such high levels of uncertainty and stress. They may also want to re-evaluate the information from the perspective of having completed the operation, or they may want answers to questions they develop after the outpatient visit [16]. For these people, information beyond typical discharge instructions must be available after surgery. This can be accomplished by using written materials in addition to verbal consultation. Preoperative information materials may be the only hospital contact a patient has once all postoperative consultations are completed, and patients may refer to them repeatedly over time while making sense of the experience [15]. Bearing this in mind, any written materials that are delivered before surgery should be prepared with the understanding that different patients may reference them once or several times, before, directly after or significantly after the event itself. It may also be useful to deliver further information after the operation, as patient recall of information provided prior to surgery – even if it is in writing – is not necessarily accurate [17].

Information delivery must also be flexible over long treatment periods, as individuals who accumulate multiple illnesses may require different levels of information as they become sicker.

Conclusion

Sociological analysis: the social meanings of being a patient

This chapter presents a conceptual framework for interpreting treatment experiences for patients. The framework features three main forms of participation: those who agree to act to fix the problem, those who accept the need to act but are dealing with the problem with strain, and those who initiate action.

These participation forms characterise the roles that people adopt when they undergo treatment as well as their relationship with doctors. The patient's role has three aspects: the participation/action style, the patient's relationship to information and the way in which the patient exercises

Table 6.1 Conceptual framework: social meanings of being a patient.

	Patient initiates action	**Patient agrees to act**	**Patient accepts need to act**
PATIENT'S ROLE			
Participation/action style	*Initiation/already* Initiates or seizes an opportunity for treatment	*Agreement/readiness* Action preferred over deliberation	*Acceptance/readying* Strain is a major feature and is evident in heightened fear, sense of burden, silence, making complaints
Relationship to information	Information important to personal control	Informed according to need	Heightened need for information of various kinds or from different sources
How patient exercises authority	Asserts symptoms, initiates treatment or investigation, seizes opportunities	Assesses illness state and symptoms	Uncertainty, ambivalence, resistance rather than an exercise in authority
PATIENT-DOCTOR RELATIONS			
Character of patient–doctor relationship	*Independent relations,* both praising and critical	*Ease of relations* Sense of shared task and responsibility	*Strain in relations and communication* No sense of shared task
Patient's perception of medical authority	Not in awe of medical authority	Works for benefit of the patient Neither oppressive nor challenged	May be oppressive May be uncertainty whether working for patient's benefit
Patient's trust of medical authority	Has to be earned through egalitarian interactions and technical competence Mistrust may lead the patient to challenge authority	Has to be earned through egalitarian interactions and technical competence Positive experience strongly linked to feelings of trust and confidence	Trust withheld May express denial at medical assessment, may seek second opinion
Personal meaning	*Personal meaning* arises from intersection of social life (personal history, prior illness); physical experience of treatment; and knowledge of medical information and practice		
Participation transformation	Participation forms, patterns and roles are *transformed* by changing circumstances, such as accumulation of illness		

authority. The patient's relationship with doctors is comprised by the character of the doctor–patient interaction and the patient's perception of and trust in medical authority. Two features of the conceptual framework (see Table 6.1) apply to all patients: personal meaning of the treatment experience and participation transformation.

Surgery is a unique experience and a prism through which we can learn more of how people interact and participate in health and health treatment. Qualitative research using in-depth interviews helps to illuminate the patient experience, informing the development of new communication models.

References

1. Hill S (2003) The Social Meanings of Being a Patient: A Sociological Analysis of the Experience of Surgery [PhD]. La Trobe University, Bundoora.
2. Coulter A, Ellins J (2007) Effectiveness of strategies for informing, educating, and involving patients. *British Medical Journal* **335**, 24–27.
3. Lustria ML, Cortese J, Noar SM, Glueckauf RL (2009) Computer-tailored health interventions delivered over the web: review and analysis of key components. *Patient Education and Counseling* **74**, 156–173.
4. Charles C, Gafni A, Whelan T (1997) Shared decision-making in the medical encounter: what does it mean? (Or it takes at least two to tango). *Social Science & Medicine* **44**, 681–692.
5. Makoul G, Clayman ML (2006) An integrative model of shared decision making in medical encounters. *Patient Education and Counseling* **60**, 301–312.
6. Edwards A, Elwyn G (2009) *Shared Decision-Making in Health Care: Achieving Evidence-Based Patient Choice*. Oxford University Press, Oxford.
7. Joosten E, DeFuentes-Merillas L, de Weert G (2008) Systematic review of the effects of shared decision-making on patient satisfaction: treatment adherence and health status. *Psychotherapy & Psychosomatics* **77**, 219–226.
8. Kinnersley P, Edwards A, Hood K, et al. (2007) Interventions before consultations for helping patients address their information needs. *Cochrane Database of Systematic Reviews*, CD004565.
9. Stewart MA (1995) Effective physician-patient communication and health outcomes: a review. *Canadian Medical Association Journal* **152**, 1423–1433.
10. Pagano M (2010) *Interactive Case Studies in Health Communication*. Jones and Bartlett Publishers, Sudbury.
11. Mauleon AL, Palo-Bengtsson L, Ekman SL (2007) Patients experiencing local anaesthesia and hip surgery. *Journal of Clinical Nursing* **16**, 892–899.
12. Klafta JM, Roizen MF (1996) Current understanding of patients' attitudes toward and preparation for anesthesia: a review. *Anesthesia and Analgesia* **83**, 1314–1321.
13. McCarthy R, Trigg R, John C, Gough M, Horrocks M (2004) Patient satisfaction for carotid endarterectomy performed under local anaesthesia. *European Journal of Vascular and Endovascular Surgery* **27**, 654–659.
14. Davies MJ, Silbert BS, Scott DA, Cook RJ, Mooney PH, Blyth C (1997) Superficial and deep cervical plexus block for carotid artery surgery: a prospective study of 1000 blocks. *Regional Anesthesia* **22**, 442–446.

15. Walker JA (2007) What is the effect of preoperative information on patient satisfaction? *British Journal of Nursing* **16**, 27–32.
16. Tang PC, Newcomb C (1998) Informing patients: a guide for providing patient health information. *Journal of the American Medical Informatics Association* **5**, 563–570.
17. Middleton S, Gattellari M, Harris JP, Ward JE (2006) Assessing surgeons' disclosure of risk information before carotid endarterectomy. *ANZ Journal of Surgery* **76**, 618–624.

CHAPTER 7

Disclosure: a case study of communication about medically acquired risk for a rare disease

Rebecca E. Ryan[1], *Jessica Kaufman*[2] *and Sophie Hill*[3]
[1]Research Fellow, Cochrane Consumers and Communication Review Group, Centre for Health Communication and Participation, Australian Institute for Primary Care and Ageing, La Trobe University, Bundoora, Victoria, Australia
[2]Research Officer, Cochrane Consumers and Communication Review Group, Centre for Health Communication and Participation, Australian Institute for Primary Care and Ageing, La Trobe University, Bundoora, Victoria, Australia
[3]Coordinating Editor/Head, Cochrane Consumers and Communication Review Group, Centre for Health Communication and Participation, Australian Institute for Primary Care and Ageing, La Trobe University, Bundoora, Victoria, Australia

Introduction

Implicit in an evidence-informed approach to health communication is the understanding that communication interventions can be done well or poorly and can have positive or negative effects and that these effects can be evaluated. Careful analysis of interventions can help inform a communication strategy that minimises harm and negative outcomes.

Communicating with consumers about a disease or disease risk is a sensitive undertaking, especially when exposure has occurred during the course of medical treatment. Poor communication strategies relating to a disease risk can lead to confusion, psychological harm and other negative effects. This chapter examines the notification and ongoing communication following an adverse medical event in a case study of the risk of Creutzfeldt–Jakob disease (CJD) acquired through medical treatment. Drawing from all available sources, including the stories of consumers

The Knowledgeable Patient: Communication and Participation in Health – A Cochrane Handbook, First Edition.
Edited by Sophie Hill.

and carers, we outline the findings of a systematic review and present a framework identifying how communication might best happen in these situations.

Communication and disclosure about adverse events

Transparency in communication is becoming increasingly important in healthcare, particularly as the patient's role shifts from passive participant to active consumer. Healthcare providers and systems have an ethical imperative to respect the patient's right to know about issues and events that affect their care. This includes open disclosure following adverse events.

Adverse events are incidents in which a patient experiences unintended harm while receiving medical treatment [1]. Adverse events are not necessarily due to medical errors, and in some cases, the cause of the event may be difficult to ascertain. A variety of incidents that cause harm may be categorised as adverse events: some may be due to treatment (e.g. prescribing or administering the wrong medicine or dosage), they may be known risks of a procedure (e.g. complications of a surgery or therapy) or they may be indirectly related to treatment (e.g. healthcare-acquired infection or exposure to a disease or disease risk).

Notifying people of such incidents is in line with recent moves to support health services in disclosing information related to adverse incidents that occur while receiving medical care [2, 3]. Under a policy of open disclosure, the patient must be informed of the harm that has occurred regardless of its cause.

Communication following adverse events is especially sensitive and challenging. Doctors may be reluctant to apologise or inform patients that mistakes have occurred, as it may be seen as an admission of culpability and could raise liability concerns [4, 5]. Patients may suffer secondary harms, such as confusion, anxiety or distress, if poor communication strategies are used when disclosing information about adverse events, such as exposure to a disease risk [6]. Internationally, health safety organisations are moving to establish broad standards for communication strategies to ensure that adverse event disclosure occurs in a consistent and respectful manner (e.g. Canada [7], Australia [8] and the United Kingdom [9]). These documents provide a background against which communication strategies and programmes could be developed, outlining timelines for disclosure, who should deliver the information, where disclosure should occur and what should be included in the communication.

Why was the research conducted?

Risk for a rare disease: the case of CJD

In 2006, the Cochrane Consumers and Communication Review Group (CC&CRG) began a systematic review of the evidence on strategies for notifying and supporting people who have been exposed to CJD risk through medical treatment. This chapter is based on this comprehensive systematic review, which is available online as a report [6]. The systematic review collected evidence from all sources, including people's experiences, needs and preferences, and used qualitative methods to synthesise this evidence. The CC&CRG is also undertaking a Cochrane review on this same topic, the protocol of which is available online [10].

CJD is a very rare disease, and little is known about people's needs and preferences for notification of risk and support after notification. Before the CC&CRG systematic review, the existing research evidence in this area had never been systematically assembled and assessed to identify the main themes of people's experiences and preferences for communication and support.

CJD and its variant form – variant CJD (vCJD) – are rare, fatal, neurodegenerative diseases with very long incubation periods. While CJD can occur spontaneously or genetically, this review focused on the medically acquired forms of the disease.

CJD can be transmitted through a small number of specific medical procedures, such as brain surgery and human pituitary hormone treatment. vCJD is most often acquired by consuming contaminated meat, but it can also be spread medically through blood transfusions [6].

To protect public health, it may often be necessary to inform people when they may have been exposed to CJD or vCJD risk. Additional infection control measures may be needed, such as preventing people at CJD or vCJD risk from donating blood or undergoing certain healthcare procedures without additional infection control measures in place [8].

There are several features unique to these diseases that make communication about exposure to risk very challenging. There is no screening test for CJD or vCJD, and they are resistant to medical sterilisation techniques, which means that people receiving certain types of surgery may be treated with potentially infected equipment from a previous patient. This happens in a *very* small number of cases, but it is possible. The period between infection and presentation of symptoms can be as long as several decades. This lengthy incubation period means that the risk may not be identified until many years later when an individual develops what is determined to be CJD or vCJD. At that point, the individual's medical history must be traced backwards and anyone who may have been exposed to the risk of infection must be notified. In some cases, hundreds of people may need to be contacted.

With no way to test for exposure to CJD or vCJD, potentially infected individuals can be told only that they have an increased risk of developing symptoms, relative to the rest of the population, at some uncertain time in the future. The seriousness of the disease and the uncertainty of the risk for future disease can make notification a highly distressing event, which may cause significant anxiety and psychological harm. It may also lead to future problems such as discrimination in accessing healthcare for people who are deemed to be 'at risk' for CJD or vCJD.

For these reasons, communication related to CJD and vCJD risk must be carefully considered. The information must be conveyed in a way that causes the least harm to individuals and their families.

What consumers said was important

Notification of exposure to CJD or vCJD risk can have far-reaching negative consequences, so it is imperative that health services employ the best communication and support practices for people at risk. However, exactly what constitutes these best practices is not clear. Research in this area is fragmented and has not been compiled and assessed systematically to determine the different possible methods of communication with people at risk or the impacts of such communication. Some questions that should be considered when developing risk communication strategies include the following:

- What method should be used for notification, and by whom should it be carried out?
- What format or approach is most effective, and how should it be staged or timed?
- What training or resources are needed to implement the communication strategy?

It is also important to consider the need for ongoing communication and support, particularly for those at risk for a disease such as CJD or vCJD which may play a continuing and changing role throughout a person's life.

While rigorous research is often based on controlled trials, important conclusions can also be drawn from accounts of people's experiences, needs and preferences. This type of information is valuable particularly when assessing and improving communication and support strategies. For rare diseases in particular, controlled research designs may not be possible or suitable to answer all questions. The rationale for the CC&CRG research, which was broad and looked at all available forms of evidence, was to gather as much information as possible to inform communication strategies for CJD and vCJD risk.

What people want: assessing needs and preferences

When an adverse event has occurred in healthcare, people generally want to be informed [4, 11]. Even with the current increasing emphasis on open disclosure, there are indications that many adverse events remain unreported, and historically, this was often the case [4, 5, 11]. Several studies of people's preferences for disclosure indicate that communication should contain detailed information, explaining the event, how it will affect them, what steps are being taken to prevent future occurrences of the same problem and, significantly, an expression of regret. People also want access to ongoing emotional support [4, 11].

Research suggests that people exposed to CJD or vCJD risk have very similar needs and preferences to those affected by other types of adverse events. People at risk, in general, would prefer to be notified of their risk status even if it is distressing [6, 12–14]. People also want ongoing information and support.

How to inform people – the best *method* of disclosure – is less certain. There has been limited rigorous research into the most preferred communication medium for notifying people of their risk for CJD or vCJD. Data from surveys of people at risk suggest that if presented with the choice of notification via letter, telephone call or consultation, people may prefer a telephone call the least.

However, all three methods may be potentially harmful if not carried out appropriately, and there may not be a single best fit for all people at risk [6]. For instance, research on people at risk for CJD or vCJD suggests that people receiving risk information for the first time by telephone or in a consultation may experience harm or be at a disadvantage because they have not had a chance to prepare for the news or formulate questions. If they are told only verbally without supporting written materials, they may have difficulty understanding and recalling information due to the shock of the situation. It may be that the best method of disclosure would be a combination technique: a letter followed by a consultation, for instance.

People generally prefer to be notified by their general practitioner (GP) or another familiar healthcare professional, rather than a professional who is unknown to them [15, 16].

Further research into notification strategies should include input from those at risk and their families to determine the most effective and sensitive communication techniques.

What people do not want: assessing harms

The goal of risk communication in the case of CJD or vCJD risk is to minimise harm caused to people and their carers while effectively communicating information about the risk. Unavoidable harms are those which arise due to the *content* of the communication, such as the long-term uncertainty associated with CJD and vCJD risk and the fatal and untreatable nature of the disease. The impact of these harms may be ameliorated by the provision of support services following notification.

Avoidable harms are those associated with the *method* of the communication. Poor communication strategies that are piecemeal, accidental, disorganised, impersonal or delayed can cause serious harm to individuals and their families [4]. People who learn of their risk status through organ donation checks, blood transfusion screening or preoperative screening, for example, may be vulnerable to harmful effects including psychological trauma and family disruption. These harms could be avoided with better planning, coordination and sensitivity of the notification.

Generally, people find notification less acceptable if the person notifying them is not knowledgeable about CJD and vCJD risk, if they deviate from the planned timing or process for disclosure or if the person at risk has to look elsewhere for information after they have been notified. Other less preferred features of notification include inadequate follow-up or support and learning about at-risk status from the media [6].

One of the most tangible and disturbing harms suffered by people at risk is the stigma and associated healthcare discrimination that arises from their at-risk status. Because healthcare professionals may have limited or incorrect information regarding CJD and vCJD risk, people at risk can experience delays and rejections when seeking treatment [6]. Communication and education about CJD and vCJD risk should reach beyond the person at risk to include health professionals and the community in order to reduce this discrimination.

Implications of the findings: a framework for evidence-informed communication for people at risk

We systematically looked at the research on the experiences, preferences and needs of people at risk and thematically analysed it to develop a framework to inform how communication might best be carried out when people are exposed to CJD or vCJD risk via medical treatment [6]. The major theme of the communication framework is the need for a standardised, planned approach to notification and support, as opposed to ad hoc or disconnected communication events.

Practically, this requires a series of coordinated, interrelated communication processes as well as appropriate support and educational structures for individuals at risk and other groups including healthcare professionals, the public and the media. For an illustration of the communication framework proposed, see Figure 7.1.

The framework is fundamentally patient centred, meaning that all decisions and actions should be flexible and responsive to the needs of the person at risk and their family. It is broken down into several major interrelated sections, each with specific aims involving different communication processes. The four major sections of the framework are outlined below.

1. National communication policy

There should be an overarching national standard for all communication related to CJD and vCJD risk so that when incidents occur in healthcare settings, people know what to do and how to respond. This policy should establish a standardised process for notifying people that they may be at risk and updating people whose at-risk status changes through further

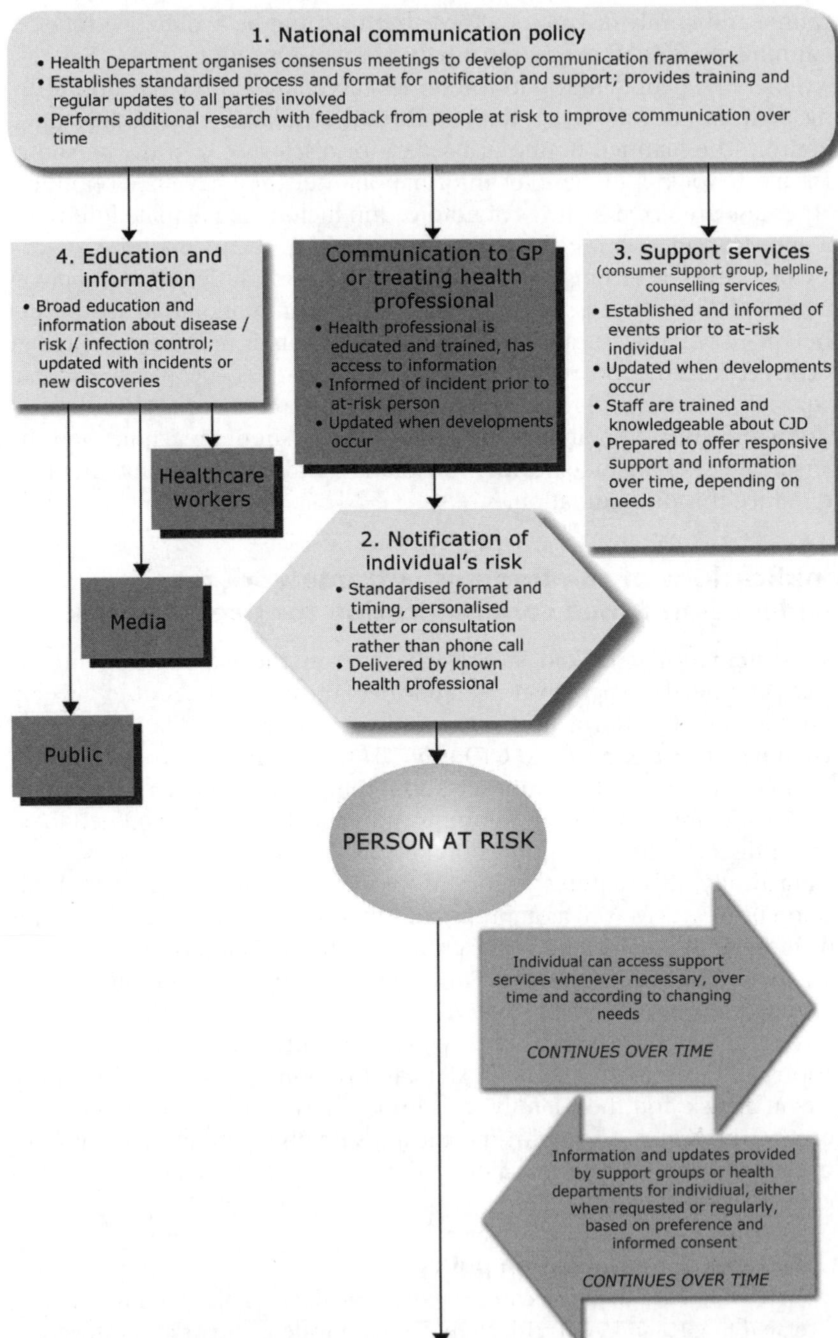

Figure 7.1 Major components of the framework for communicating with people about CJD or vCJD risk.

discoveries. Much like the national open-disclosure policies described earlier, this communication policy should outline how and when to inform, who delivers the information and what is said. This may limit the potentially harmful effects of notification.

Communication strategies should be developed through meetings involving policy makers, healthcare workers, experts and, particularly, consumers from CJD-affected groups. Additional research should be conducted, seeking feedback from people at risk to determine the long-term social and psychological effects of living with risk, the best formats for risk notification and what people need in terms of ongoing support.

Other responsibilities of a national communication policy include protecting the confidentiality of people at risk, monitoring healthcare access to ensure no discrimination occurs and recognising the need for an ongoing and supportive relationship with people at risk and their families.

2. Notification

Notification must be planned and deliberate and must consider the impact of the information. It must ensure that people receive the best possible care and that communication happens in a manner that causes the least anxiety and distress.

Notification should be standardised in form and timing, personalised wherever possible, and clearly and concisely stated. It should acknowledge the uncertainty of risk and explain the rationale for the notification (protection of public health).

The person delivering the information (in most cases, the individual's GP or another healthcare professional) should be someone the individual knows, rather than an unfamiliar healthcare professional. The informant should be trained and knowledgeable about the disease and should offer access to further information and support. Even if the individual's GP is not involved in the notification itself, they must be educated about CJD and risk and notified in advance, and should be available to provide information, ongoing support and consultations to the person at risk if they would like it.

Although the research into the best format for notification is not conclusive, it suggests that being told by telephone may be the method that people favour least. A letter or consultation, or a combination of these two, may be the preferred method. This issue needs further research.

3. Support

People at risk need ongoing access to trained and knowledgeable support services, which must be able to respond to the changing needs of the at-risk community.

Support networks, including consumer support groups and counselling services, must be in place and informed before any notification of individuals occurs. Whenever a new incident occurs, such as a new identification of risk or the death of an at-risk individual from CJD, the support network must be informed before people are notified to ensure readiness to provide support.

Because the needs of individuals are likely to change over time, support services must be available on a long-term basis and should be responsive to these changes, taking into account the effect of new discoveries and incidents upon the needs of individuals.

Wherever possible, support should be tailored to the needs and desires of the individual. For instance, one person might want regular updates on new or emerging information about CJD and vCJD provided to them by newsletter, while another may wish to receive information only when he or she contacts a support group with specific queries. All information provided should be understandable, easily accessible and accurate. It should also be up to date.

4. Education and information

Many different groups must be educated and informed about CJD and risk. This communication should also be standardised, because it can affect the well-being of the individual in direct and indirect ways.

Health professionals must be educated about CJD, risk and infection control guidelines. They should be made aware of the communication protocols and the potential negative impact of poor notification strategies.

Consumer support groups must be informed when incidents and developments occur. These groups in turn should raise awareness of their activities and functions to enable those at risk to access support.

Public communication should include community education and referral to further information and support. Greater public understanding and awareness may reduce discrimination of people at risk.

Communication with the *media* should emphasise sensitivity to those at risk. When incidents occur, individuals should hear of them through the appropriate personalised channel, rather than from a media outlet. Members of the media should be educated to avoid the perception that CJD is caused by medical negligence.

Discussion and conclusions

The experience of a rare disease

Although rare diseases are a highly heterogeneous group of conditions, they are often researched and discussed as a single category, defined by their rarity rather than shared clinical features. There are obvious limits to the parallels that can be drawn between different diseases, but the experiences of people receiving CJD or vCJD risk notification have much in common with those of people dealing with the diagnosis of other rare diseases.

The European Organisation for Rare Diseases (EURORDIS) [17] recently conducted an in-depth survey addressing issues surrounding rare diseases and their diagnosis, notification and treatment experiences for patients. The survey found that poor notification practices were a significant problem, with 35% of respondents indicating that they were informed of their diagnosis in a poor or unacceptable manner or situation. The EURORDIS survey also revealed that people dealing with rare diseases often encounter delays in receiving care or must seek care from multiple doctors, leading to a loss of confidence in the health system as a whole. This survey showed that nearly one in five respondents was rejected by a healthcare professional, most often because of the complexity of their disease and/or symptoms.

A qualitative study based on interviews with patients with rare diseases reiterated these points [18]. People with rare diseases encounter many medical challenges even before they have been diagnosed, such as periods of diagnostic uncertainty and lack of, or incorrect, treatment. However, respondents for this study were largely accepting of these problems and agreed that their greatest criticism was not with the practice of medicine but with the communication related to their disease. The participants were highly critical of health professionals who were poorly informed about the disease, who did not respect the concerns of the patients and their families, and who delivered the diagnosis in an inappropriate or upsetting manner.

People with a *risk* for a rare disease – CJD or vCJD – report similar experiences to those *diagnosed* with a rare disease. The unique and isolated nature of individual rare diseases can make it difficult to recognise that a problem may be systemic rather than specific, but when taken together, the findings of this research suggest that the communication problems in these scenarios may be characteristic of rare diseases in general. As such, it may be possible to develop communication strategies that are applicable to individuals across different rare diseases. The views of those living with a rare disease or the risk of a rare disease indicate that communication strategies should be better planned and coordinated, with an ongoing and patient-centred focus in order to improve people's health outcomes and experiences of healthcare.

Conclusion

People exposed to CJD or vCJD risk through medical treatment may need to be notified of their risk in order to protect the public health, but evidence-based communication indicates that there are both effective and harmful ways to do this. Poor and ad hoc communication strategies can cause negative health outcomes for any person receiving notification after an adverse medical event or a diagnosis of a rare disease. Our systematic analysis of the experiences, needs and preferences of people at risk for CJD or vCJD informed a patient-centred communication framework that considered the impact of this information [6]. People at risk should receive communication that is sensitive and appropriate, with ongoing support that changes with their needs. The wider context of health professionals, policy makers, the public and the media should also be included in this communication strategy, with a particular focus on eliminating stigma and healthcare discrimination.

References

1. Australian Council for Safety and Quality in Health Care (2003) *Open Disclosure Standard: A National Standard for Open Communication in Public and Private Hospitals, Following an Adverse Event in Health Care*. Australian Council for Safety and Quality in Health Care. Available from: http://www.safetyandquality.gov.au/internet/safety/publishing.nsf/Content/a-zpublicationsm-o/$File/OpenDisclosure_web.pdf http://www.safetyandquality.gov.au/internet/safety/publishing.nsf/Content/3B994EFC1C9C0B22CA25741F0019FDEE/$File/NOD-Std reprinted 2008.pdf. Accessed: 19 October 2010.
2. Iedema R, Sorensen R, Manias E, et al. (2008) Patients' and family members' experiences of open disclosure following adverse events. *International Journal for Quality in Health Care* **20**, 421–432.
3. Mazor KM, Simon SR, Gurwitz JH (2004) Communicating with patients about medical errors: a review of the literature. *Archives of Internal Medicine* **164**, 1690–1697.
4. Gallagher TH, Waterman AD, Ebers AG, Fraser VJ, Levinson W (2003) Patients' and physicians' attitudes regarding the disclosure of medical errors. *Journal of the American Medical Association* **289**, 1001–1007.
5. Chafe R, Levinson W, Sullivan T (2009) Disclosing errors that affect multiple patients. *Canadian Medical Association Journal* **180**, 1125–1127.
6. Ryan R, Lowe D, Hill S, Mead C (2008) *Evidence on Strategies for Notifying and Supporting Consumers Following Exposure to the Risk of Creutzfeldt-Jakob Disease (CJD) Through Medical Treatment: A Review of the Evidence: A Report to the Department of Human Services Victoria*. Available from: http://www.health.vic.gov.au/consumer/pubs/notifying_cjd.htm. Accessed: 3 March 2010.
7. Canadian Patient Safety Institute (2008) *Canadian Disclosure Guidelines*. Canadian Patient Safety Institute, Ottawa. Available from: http://www.patientsafetyinstitute.ca/English/toolsResources/disclosure/Documents/CPSI%20-%20Canadian%20Disclosure%20Guidlines%20English.pdf. Accessed: 2 March 2010.
8. Australian Government Department of Health and Ageing (2007) Chapter 31 Creutzfeldt-Jakob disease. In: *Infection Control Guidelines for the Prevention of Transmission of Infectious Diseases in the Health Care Setting: Part 4 Managing Infectious Diseases in the Health Care Setting*. Available from: http://www.health.gov.au/internet/main/publishing.nsf/Content/icg-guidelines-index.htm. Accessed: 28 July 2008.

9. National Patient Safety Agency (2009) *Being Open: Communicating Patient Safety Incidents With Patients, Their Families and Carers*. The Agency, London. Available from: http://www.nrls.npsa.nhs.uk/EasySiteWeb/getresource.axd?AssetID=65172&type=full&servicetype=Attachment. Accessed: 3 March 2010.
10. Ryan R, Hill S, Lowe D, Allen K, Taylor M, Mead C (2011) Notification and support for people exposed to the risk of Creutzfeldt-Jakob disease (CJD) (or other prion diseases) through medical treatment (iatrogenically). *Cochrane Database of Systematic Reviews*, CD007578.
11. Levinson W (2009) Disclosing medical errors to patients: a challenge for health care professionals and institutions. *Patient Education and Counseling* **76**, 296–299.
12. Blajchman MA, Goldman M, Webert KE, Vamvakas EC, Hannon J, Delage G (2004) Proceedings of a consensus conference: the screening of blood donors for variant CJD. *Transfusion Medicine Reviews* **18**, 73–92.
13. Hewitt PE (2004) Implications of notifying donors and recipients. *Vox Sanguinis* **87(**Suppl. 2), 1–2.
14. Larke B (1998) The quandary of Creutzfeldt-Jakob disease. *Journal of the Canadian Medical Association* **159**, 789–791.
15. Hewitt PE, Moore C, Soldan K (2006) vCJD donor notification exercise: 2005. *Clinical Ethics* **1**, 172–178.
16. vCJD Clinical Governance Advisory Group (2007) *vCJD Clinical Governance Advisory Group Report: An Independent Review for the Department of Health*. Available from: www.dh.gov.uk. Accessed: 28 January 2008.
17. European Organisation for Rare Diseases (2009) *The Voice of 12,000 Patients: Experiences and Expectations of Rare Disease Patients on Diagnosis and Care in Europe. A report based on the EurordisCare2 and EurordisCare3 Surveys*. Available from: http://www.eurordis.org/IMG/pdf/voice_12000_patients/EURORDISCARE_FULLBOOKr.pdf. Accessed: 16 March 2010.
18. Huyard C (2009) What, if anything, is specific about having a rare disorder? Patients' judgements on being ill and being rare. *Health Expectations* **12**, 361–370.

CHAPTER 8

How I used a systematic review from *The Cochrane Library*

Helen Dilkes[1], Jessica Kaufman[2] and Sophie Hill[3]
[1]Research Officer, Health Knowledge Network, Centre for Health Communication and Participation, Australian Institute for Primary Care and Ageing, La Trobe University, Bundoora, Victoria, Australia
[2]Research Officer, Cochrane Consumers and Communication Review Group, Centre for Health Communication and Participation, Australian Institute for Primary Care and Ageing, La Trobe University, Bundoora, Victoria, Australia
[3]Coordinating Editor/Head, Cochrane Consumers and Communication Review Group, Centre for Health Communication and Participation, Australian Institute for Primary Care and Ageing, La Trobe University, Bundoora, Victoria, Australia

Why was the research conducted?

There is a long recorded history in research indicating that patients want more information than they receive. For instance, 40 years of large Australian and British studies document patients' expressed desire for more information than they were given [1–8] (see Chapter 6).

Surgical patients, for example, report that they want information about a wide range of topics and issues. This includes information about the illness, treatment, risks and prognosis, also about what to anticipate, ways they can look after themselves, find information, support and other services, and make better use of their consultations with doctors [6–10].

Increasingly, clinicians are using evidence from systematic reviews of controlled trials to stay abreast of the latest research and inform their practice [11] and to contribute to the process of shared decision-making with their patients [12]. This process is facilitated by initiatives in medical education, decision tools and the provision of rigorous, up-to-date syntheses of the evidence in systematic reviews.

A major source of evidence from systematic reviews is *The Cochrane Library*. Cochrane reviews are high-quality syntheses of the results of

The Knowledgeable Patient: Communication and Participation in Health – A Cochrane Handbook, First Edition.
Edited by Sophie Hill.

controlled trials of clinical, behavioural, educational and organisational interventions to improve health [13, 14]. They are developed using rigorous methods to reduce bias [15]. Their final published form includes the full review, abstract, lay summary and detailed tables. They are kept up to date as new trials emerge.

Health information derived from these sources is simultaneously being made available to the public. In Australia, a key vehicle for this to occur is through the internet, facilitated by a nationally funded subscription to *The Cochrane Library* (www.thecochranelibrary.com) or via government websites such as *HealthInsite* (www.healthinsite.gov.au). Government commitment to improving access to sources of evidence rests on research that has shown that information improves people's knowledge, capacity to manage their health and health literacy [16, 17].

The Cochrane Library is a unique and complex resource for health professionals and consumers, but its use depends on people understanding the concepts and methods of systematic reviews, i.e. the science behind the review. Recent testing of users' experiences of using and finding information in *The Cochrane Library* indicates problems of inaccessible material and technical language hindering understanding [16]. There has been research into how to present summary formats of research-based information clearly and unambiguously [17, 18]. However, this research showed that consumers want information that is relevant to their situation, in language and using terminology they can understand and from a source they can trust.

Little research has been done with consumers and carers about how they are using evidence. This led to the qualitative research described in this chapter. Four participants – Molly, Emma, Isobelle and Adam – were involved in a focus group in Melbourne in 2009, recalling and talking about how, why and when they consulted *The Cochrane Library*, what they found, how they felt about it and how it helped them think about and/or make decisions about their healthcare. Ethics Committee approval from La Trobe University was granted for the study, and the names of the participants have been changed. All participants knew about *The Cochrane Library* and Cochrane reviews before the start of the project. This means that compared with new or occasional users, they were highly research-literate participants. Analysis of the transcripts is presented first and Molly's story is threaded throughout and gives the perspective of a parent seeking information on evidence for and against surgery for her son.

What consumers said was important

When people consulted a Cochrane review

Individual information-seeking strategies and situations varied. For instance, Adam went looking for evidence at the end of the information-seeking process, to confirm what was found elsewhere. Emma looked for information after seeing a surgeon, to see if she fitted into the scenario for surgery (participant age for example). And Isobelle, who had a chronic illness, checked regularly between doctor/specialist visits just in case something relevant had been published.

Molly's story:

> It was for a family member, for my son ... it was a decision my husband and I had to make. My son had recurrent ear infections and he previously had grommets ... one of them had fallen out and the other one had scarred and wasn't working any more ... and he had had lots more ear infections and his hearing was down as a result of it.
>
> We just wanted a little bit more information after seeing the surgeon. So we did consult *The Cochrane Library*. [Molly knew about The Library but had not thought to look but her husband suggested a Google search with 'Cochrane' in combination with Glue ear and grommets ... and it came up with three reviews that were quite relevant.]

Sections of a review which are useful

Participants discussed how they went into each review in detail – looking deeper than simply reading the 'bottom line' of the conclusions. One reported that the title was informative because it lets readers know if it is relevant to them and because it contains key information about the participants in the trial and the intervention. This is because Cochrane reviews follow standard formats (intervention for health problem). Another talked of reading the background section, which sets up the rationale for the review.

Participants knew the difference between a Cochrane protocol (the formal plan for a review, which is published on *The Cochrane Library*) and a Cochrane review (the completed analysis). They also went looking for individual studies to see if the people in the trials were similar in social background, sex and age. One looked at the plain language summary first, then the background, and then the statistical analyses, called forest plots (see Table 8.1 for an explanation of the standard components of all Cochrane reviews, using Gareth Hollands and colleagues' 2010 Cochrane review to illustrate key components as outlined in the *Cochrane Handbook* [15,19]).

Molly's story:

> [One of the reasons for looking further for evidence-based information was that] we weren't sure whether he really did fit the scenario. He had had multiple ear infections but we weren't sure whether that was normal as well. So one of the things that we found very useful from the Cochrane Review was in the Background section – it describes what is an acute condition for ear infections and it was useful because it confirmed for us that it was three or more infections over a six month period or four over a year and he had had a lot more.

Table 8.1 Elements of a Cochrane review.

Basic review information *(freely available to all online throughout the world)*	
Title	Standardised format that succinctly states the focus of the review: [Intervention] for [health problem] Example: *Visual feedback of individuals' medical imaging results for changing health behaviour*
Abstract	Brief summary of the review, divided into sections that correspond to those in the main review
Plain language summary	Summary paragraph that explains the review in a straightforward style that can be understood by consumers
Detailed review information *(available with an institutional or national subscription)*	
Background	Introduction to the context and significance of the question being asked in the review Example: *Feedback of medical imaging results can reveal visual evidence of actual bodily harm attributable to a given behaviour. This may offer a particularly promising approach to motivating changes in health behaviour to decrease risk*
Objectives	Short description of the primary aim of the review Example: *To assess the extent to which feedback to individuals of images of their own bodies created during medical imaging procedures increases or decreases a range of health behaviours*
Selection criteria	Description of the features of the studies under consideration in the review Example: **Types of studies** – *randomised or quasi-randomised controlled trials* **Types of participants** – *adult non-pregnant individuals undergoing medical imaging procedures* **Types of interventions** – *presentation and explanation of an individual's medical imaging results* **Types of outcome measures** – *behavioural outcomes measured by questionnaire and self-report (dietary behaviour, physical activity, smoking, alcohol consumption, etc.)*
Search strategy	Specific explanation of how searches for relevant information were conducted, including details of accessed databases, journals, conference proceedings, etc. Example: *We searched the Cochrane Central Register of Controlled Trials, MEDLINE, EMBASE, CINAHL, PsycINFO and reference lists of articles*

(Continued)

Table 8.1 (*Continued*)

Methods of the review	Details on what was done to obtain the results of the review Example: *Methods used to identify relevant studies* *Criteria used to assess quality of included studies* *Data extraction and analysis methods*
Results	What do the data show? The results may be accompanied by a graph called a forest plot to show meta-analysis. The results section has three main sections which are described below
Description of studies	Characteristics of included and excluded studies Example: *How many studies were found?* *What interventions and outcomes were examined?* *What were their inclusion criteria?* *How many participants were involved?*
Methodological quality of included studies	Assessment of risk of bias due to study quality or reporting
Effects of intervention	Summary of the findings of the review. These should directly address the review objectives rather than list the findings of each study Example: *There was a statistically significant increase in smoking cessation behaviours with the intervention . . . indicating that the odds of participants allocated to the interventions engaging in smoking cessation behaviours were 2.81 times that of those allocated to the control conditions*
Discussion	Interpretation and assessment of the results
Author's conclusions	Brief, practical information divided into two categories: implications for practice and implications for research
Figures	Graphical presentation of the results and other information
Tables	Additional information organised into tables, the most important being characteristics of included studies (a structured summary of each individual trial)

How the Cochrane review helped

The information in reviews commonly confirmed what had been found elsewhere or what had been told to them. Participants talked about a range of ways in which the information was helpful. It backed up the decision to have an operation and informed its timing. Reviews provided information on different sorts of health outcomes, such as effects on pain, quality of life or side effects of medicines. Isobelle, prescribed a new medicine for a serious chronic disease, was interested in the major risks – a risk of stroke and heart attack – and weighing up these against a minor reduction in pain, chose not to take the new medicine. Some reviews may not have influenced a specific decision because there was no choice, but they provided a sense of comfort and control, reassuring the participant that all risks and benefits had been looked into. For Emma, talking about the review with her doctor led to being given more detailed information, including details of how the operation was done and the consequences of not doing anything.

Molly's story:

> And we also wanted to know what other possible interventions there might have been that we weren't aware of or hadn't considered – rather than having surgery, minor surgery, and go under anaesthetic, and he is only five. We also found that the reviews helped in terms of what other options there were, and there weren't many. There were antibiotics that he had had for each ear infection, antibiotics in an ongoing way as a prophylaxis sort of thing, and watchful waiting and we didn't want to give him antibiotics as a prophylactic, and watchful waiting we had already done. It confirmed for us that there wasn't something else we had overlooked.
>
> [Having looked at the pros and cons and talked to the surgeon, the evidence] informs us that if we were interested in him starting prep [preparatory school] we wanted him to have the best possible start, have his good hearing and not be suffering from ear infections. So in January we actually had his grommets done and it's almost six months now and he is going quite well. So it informed the timing of the decision for us as well. We could have had it done any time from when we had seen a specialist which was six months earlier, but in particular it did inform the timing.

What people hoped to find from reviews

Participants accessed *The Cochrane Library* hoping to find quality studies describing the effectiveness of certain interventions in relation to specific outcomes, but most discovered that the information available was not personally relevant enough to fully inform a decision.

Isobelle wanted to read studies specific to her condition or medications, but was frustrated by an absence of pertinent reviews. Most participants found information that was only somewhat relevant to them and used the reviews as supporting or supplementary sources of knowledge rather than personal decision-making tools. Adam, for instance, performed extensive research elsewhere before accessing the Library in order to confirm what he had already learned. Molly was able to find reviews that helped her determine the appropriate timing for her son's intervention, but differences between her son and the study populations made it difficult to use the Library to evaluate how effective the intervention might be.

Molly's story:

> We were hoping to find out whether the intervention would be effective for the outcomes we were interested in [hearing loss, infections, behaviour] and for how long they were effective and whether there was anything we had overlooked in terms of alternative interventions ... It was useful but not perfect because of the population.

Emergent theme of people managing their own health

All the participants are active healthcare information seekers with a high level of health literacy. Isobelle's doctor says she should self-manage her health. She agrees but finds this challenging in grey areas such as deciding whether to take an additional drug. Emma said that performing her own research and gaining knowledge through *The Cochrane Library* made her feel empowered, though the reviews she read raised new questions as well.

Molly's story:

> I suspect I will continue to find Cochrane reviews useful for situating the state of the evidence on a health intervention, and providing direction for the decisions I make regarding interventions for my own health and the health of my dependants.

Implications of the findings for health professionals

Relevant research and Cochrane reviews have the potential to benefit patients by informing the care provided by health professionals and by supplementing and enhancing the knowledge and understanding of the patients themselves.

Evidence-based practice (EBP) requires that health professionals make healthcare decisions based on recent, relevant, high-quality research. According to Dawes and colleagues, healthcare not based on evidence is less effective and may even cause harm [11]. In the curriculum Dawes outlines for teaching healthcare professionals to use and recognise EBP, he highlights the criticality of showing professionals where to find research and how to interpret it.

Evidence is not always easily accessible, so training can be an important part of encouraging health professionals to use research in their practice. In a study evaluating the accessibility of *The Cochrane Library*, Rosenbaum and colleagues write of its complex and confusing structures, presenting significant hurdles to research access and understanding for health professionals. The participants in the study, all educated and with high health literacy rates, described feeling 'overwhelmed,' 'bombarded' and 'stupid' when trying to navigate *The Cochrane Library* [16].

Since the Rosenbaum study, steps have been taken to clarify *The Cochrane Library* and make it easier to find the evidence, but it is clear that patients seeking to use Cochrane reviews and research to aid in decision-making and supplement their knowledge will need assistance from their health professionals. Patients need to know where to find reviews, why they are a reliable source of health information and what type of information they can provide.

Clinicians should be up to date with the latest research from systematic reviews in order to refer patients in their practice to relevant information. They must also understand the structure of reviews and be able to explain how to reinterpret the information back to individuals. The use of knowledge translation tools and techniques during consultations may be helpful or necessary to translate information into language that patients can understand. Review results can be confusing, and patients may need an explanation of concepts such as risk of bias (in relation to individual studies) and how this relates to the overall findings of that review.

Health professionals need to know that patients value their perspective. Although patients might seek and find health information in reviews and from other sources, they depend on and value the perspective of their clinician because it is based on a wealth of practical experience. Information found through individual research can also be confusing or contradictory, as indicated by Glenton's study on the information provided by government-run online health portals. Glenton and colleagues found that health portal information is rarely supported by systematic reviews, and is frequently confusing, vague or incomplete [20]. A knowledgeable clinician can help patients sort through information they have found independently.

Shared decision-making is an important element of the doctor–patient relationship, particularly as it relates to patient participation and better communication. Health professionals should have a positive attitude towards patients who seek high-quality health information or who ask questions based on information and want to share in the decision-making process. The patient, rather than the health problem, should be the focus of any consultation and both the patient and the clinician should be in agreement about the problem and the course of action to be taken [21].

Clinicians must be able to adapt to the information needs of different patients, and to the same patient in different situations. As in the case of several of the surgery patients interviewed in Chapter 6, some individuals do not want to be informed in detail. Others require information pamphlets and several consultations to feel comfortably informed. Health

Table 8.2 Tools for health professionals and consumers.

Finding evidence	***The Cochrane Library*** The Cochrane Collaboration produces *The Cochrane Library* to 'help healthcare providers, policy makers, patients, their advocates and carers to make well-informed decisions about healthcare by preparing, maintaining and promoting the accessibility of Cochrane reviews of the effects of healthcare interventions' *The Cochrane Library* is a set of databases containing systematic reviews of evidence. The main database is the *Cochrane Database of Systematic Reviews*, which contains Cochrane reviews of interventions and protocols, Cochrane reviews of diagnostic test accuracy and Cochrane methodology reviews. Abstracts and summaries are freely available online, and countries with national licences also have access to complete reviews at no cost www.cochrane.org
Using evidence: health professionals	**Oxford Centre for Evidence-Based Medicine (CEBM)** 'Our broad aim is to develop, teach and promote evidence-based health care and provide support and resources to doctors and health care professionals to help maintain the highest standards of medicine' The CEBM provides tools for each step of the evidence-based medicine process: • Asking focused questions • Finding the evidence • Critical appraisal • Making a decision • Evaluating performance • Designing research www.cebm.net
Using evidence: consumers	**Patient Decision Aids, Ottawa Hospital Research Institute (OHRI)** The Patient Decision Aids group provides tools to help patients and health practitioners make decisions. Users can search for decision aids on different health topics 'Patient decision aids are tools that help people become involved in decision making by providing information about the options and outcomes and by clarifying personal values.' The site also provides resources for health professionals who want to develop or implement patient decision aids http://decisionaid.ohri.ca/

Note: All websites accessed 12 February 2010.

professionals may need to be trained to encourage question asking rather than seeing it as a threat to consultation length [21].

This chapter concludes with important resources for health professionals and consumers for finding and using evidence from systematic reviews in decision-making (see Table 8.2).

References

1. Cartwright A (1964) *Human Relations and Hospital Care*. Routledge & Kegan Paul, London.
2. Ley P, Spelman MS (1967) *Communicating With the Patient*. Staples Press, London.
3. Commonwealth Department of Health, Housing, Local Government and Community Services Australia (1993) *Defensive Medicine and Informed Consent. Report for the Review of Professional Indemnity Arrangements for Health Care Professionals*. Australian Government Publishing Service, Canberra.
4. United Kingdom, Audit Commission (1993) *What Seems to be the Matter: Communication Between Hospitals and Patients*. Her Majesty's Stationery Office and Audit Commission, London.
5. Draper M, Hill S (1995) *The Role of Patient Satisfaction Surveys in a National Approach to Hospital Quality Management. Report for the Commonwealth Department of Human Services and Health*. Australian Government Publishing Service, Canberra, pp. 12–21.
6. Coulter A, Entwistle V, Gilbert D (1998) *Informing Patients: An Assessment of the Quality of Patient Information Materials*. King's Fund Publishing, London.
7. Department of Human Services (DHS) Victoria (2001) *Well-Written Health Information. Stroke, Chest Pain and Cholecystectomy. Communicating With Consumers Series, Volume 2*. Department of Human Services Victoria, Melbourne.
8. Department of Human Services (DHS) Victoria (2001) *Well-Written Health Information. Menorrhagia, Mastitis and Pain Relief During Childbirth. Communicating With Consumers Series, Volume 3*. Department of Human Services Victoria, Melbourne.
9. Edwards D (1997) *Face to Face: Patient, Family and Professional Perspectives of Head and Neck Cancer Care*. King's Fund Publishing, London, pp. 35–37.
10. Moore J, Ziebland S, Kennedy S (2002) 'People sometimes react funny if they're not told enough': women's views about the risks of diagnostic laparoscopy. *Health Expectations* **5**, 302.
11. Dawes M, Summerskill W, Glasziou P, et al. (2005) Sicily statement on evidence-based practice. *BMC Medical Education* **5**, 1.
12. Elwyn G, Edwards A, Kinnersley P, Grol R (2000) Shared decision making and the concept of equipoise: the competences of involving patients in healthcare choices. *British Journal of General Practice* **50**, 1923–1932.
13. Moynihan R (2004) *Evaluating Health Services*. Milbank Memorial Fund, New York.
14. Shea B, Moher D, Graham I, Pham B, Tugwell P (2002) A comparison of the quality of Cochrane reviews and systematic reviews published in paper-based journals. *Evaluation and the Health Professions* **25**, 116–129.
15. Higgins J, Green S (eds.) (2009) *Cochrane Handbook for Systematic Reviews of Interventions Version 5.0.2*. Available from: www.cochrane-handbook.org. Accessed: 14 April 2010.
16. Rosenbaum S, Glenton C, Cracknell J (2008) User experiences of evidence-based online resources for health professionals: user testing of The Cochrane Library. *BMC Medical Informatics and Decision Making* **8**, 34.
17. Santesso N, Glenton C, Lang B (2008) Evidence that patients can understand and use? *Zeitschrift fur Evidenz Fortbildung und Qualitat im Gesundheitswesen* **102**, 493–496.
18. Santesso N, Glenton C, Nilsen ES, et al. (2008) [O01-3] Plain language summary format for Cochrane reviews: results of user testing. *16th Cochrane Colloquium*, Freiburg, 3–7 October 2008.

19. Hollands GJ, Hankins M, Marteau TM (2010) Visual feedback of individuals' medical imaging results for changing health behaviour. *Cochrane Database of Systematic Reviews*, CD007434.
20. Glenton C, Paulsen EJ, Oxman AD (2005) Portals to Wonderland: health portals lead to confusing information about the effects of health care. *BMC Medical Informatics and Decision Making* **5**, 7.
21. Kinnersley P, Edwards A, Hood K, et al. (2007) Interventions before consultations for helping patients address their information needs. *Cochrane Database of Systematic Reviews*, CD004565.

CHAPTER 9
Evidence and resources for systems decision-making: improving the experience of health and treatment

Dianne B. Lowe[1], *Sophie Hill*[2] *and Rebecca E. Ryan*[3]
[1]Research Officer, Cochrane Consumers and Communication Review Group, Centre for Health Communication and Participation, Australian Institute for Primary Care and Ageing, La Trobe University, Bundoora, Victoria, Australia
[2]Coordinating Editor/Head, Cochrane Consumers and Communication Review Group, Centre for Health Communication and Participation, Australian Institute for Primary Care and Ageing, La Trobe University, Bundoora, Victoria, Australia
[3]Research Fellow, Cochrane Consumers and Communication Review Group, Centre for Health Communication and Participation, Australian Institute for Primary Care and Ageing, La Trobe University, Bundoora, Victoria, Australia

This chapter combines two concepts in order to identify the scope and quantity of evidence for improving health and the experience of treatment. The first concept is termed evidence for health systems decision-making and the second is evidence to promote health and improve the experience of illness and treatment (shortened hereafter to health experiences).

Users of evidence and types of decision-making

Evidence on clinical treatments

Many systematic reviews are reviews of trials of clinical treatments and they provide evidence for different groups of people and different types of decisions. For instance, consumers may look on *The Cochrane Library* to see if there is any evidence of a treatment proposed by their doctor, and some of these kinds of experiences are discussed in Chapter 8. Their doctor may

The Knowledgeable Patient: Communication and Participation in Health – A Cochrane Handbook, First Edition. Edited by Sophie Hill.

have also seen the latest review and based a discussion of a treatment option on the results from the systematic review in addition to knowledge of the patient's preferences [1]. This is the basis of evidence-based medicine and evidence-based practice.

Evidence for the implementation of clinical treatments

Increasingly, though, as chapters in this book have demonstrated, the methods of systematic reviews have spread in application and there is a growing body of evidence summarising the effects of different types of interventions, not only clinical treatments but also interventions which aid the effective and efficient *implementation* of clinical care. This type of research has been termed implementation research by Eccles and colleagues [2].

Getting evidence into practice

Who, then, are the users of this type of evidence? An example will illustrate. In 2005, the USA's Commonwealth Fund released a six-country comparative survey with sicker adults. Responding to questions about hospital and discharge experiences, at least one-third of respondents in each country (Australia, Canada, Germany, New Zealand, the United Kingdom and USA) 'did not receive instructions about symptoms to watch for, did not know whom to contact with questions, or left without arrangements for follow-up care' (p. 512) [3].

Inadequate preparation for discharge is a cause of adverse events and readmission [4]. How could this problem be fixed and who would be most interested in knowing whether evidence exists on the effects of discharge planning and communication at discharge with consumers? We could put the onus on patients and families to 'implement' discharge planning, and it is certainly true that each patient or perhaps a family member accompanying the patient could ask for information at discharge. But the way this type of evidence would get into practice – to aid the implementation of effective clinical care – would be for the hospital to take responsibility for examining the evidence on discharge planning, and if effective, ensure it is implemented. Not surprisingly, the hospital would need a *system* of discharge planning, where all the important information is given to the patient and for staff to ensure the patient is safe to return home.

Health systems decision-making

In this chapter, this type of systematic review is called evidence for systems decision-making because the implementation of an effective intervention would not generally be the responsibility of an individual but would more commonly require a systems approach to its establishment or new models of care (see Chapter 2).

Evidence to improve health experiences

The second concept in this chapter builds on the first concept and asks, what is the range of interventions or strategies which would improve the way in which health and healthcare are experienced by consumers and carers? The promotion of health and the provision of responsive healthcare are not only about effective clinical care, although that is an essential ingredient. Our focus is active and informed consumers in both a clinical domain and a social domain.

Combining evidence which is implemented at a systems level with the concept of improving health and the experience of illness, it is possible to identify the key features of different types of interventions:

- The intervention will affect the way in which healthcare is planned, funded, delivered, regulated or evaluated.
- The intervention will affect the way in which consumers or health professionals interact, are educated, informed or communicated with.
- The intervention may affect the way in which the community is consulted or encouraged to participate [5].
- Implementation of the intervention may require the development of infrastructure, e.g. related systems, training and administrative support [6–7].
- The intervention may assist the implementation of clinical interventions; e.g. it may provide doctors with guidance on how to support patients to follow medical advice. Equally, it may be used to help doctors to follow clinical guidelines.
- Implementation of the intervention will require a programmatic decision-making framework, i.e., decision-making by more than one individual [5]. For example, evidence will be sought, assessed and integrated as part of a policy review process by government.
- Implementation may depend on an analysis of costs and benefits in addition to effects on clinical or health status outcomes.

Evidence to improve health experiences would therefore include interventions implemented at several levels, e.g. government policy, service delivery or organisational programme. Evidence for systems improvement may feed into different policy purposes such as developing a new policy or guideline, conducting a review or audit, as well as analysing research gaps and priorities or disseminating evidence in knowledge transfer networks (see Chapter 17).

Sources of evidence for systems decision-making

In the last two decades, there has been a substantial growth in the number of published systematic reviews, fuelled by the existence of the Cochrane Collaboration, as well as in response to need [8]. This has led in turn to the growth of special resource collections or databases of systematic reviews. The broader context for this has been the interest amongst those in government and quality improvement arenas for evidence relevant to improving the systems and delivery mechanisms of healthcare [9] and from interest by researchers and policy makers to bridge the science–practice gap [10]. Campbell and colleagues surveyed Australian policy makers and researchers, finding that research did not commonly influence a policy agenda, but did inform the content of policies.

Lavis and colleagues have identified some of the challenges of bridging the gap between research evidence and implementation. Research competes with many other factors in decision-making, and it is not surprising that decision-makers may not value research evidence as an input to the process. Research is usually complex, and it is therefore not easy to use or apply. Its relevance to specific audiences may be unclear [11]. Barriers to finding appropriate information in a timely way are numerous: lack of good searching skills, numerous sources, unclear quality of evidence and lack of time [12].

In addition, these types of interventions are often complex, including a number of interdependent or independent components [13]. For this reason it is often difficult to search for and locate evidence using routine searching strategies, such as searching with some keywords or index terms. Hand searching is the most reliable way to capture all relevant reviews, but this is far too time-consuming for most people.

Even once you have solved the problem of identifying the research, you must still do something meaningful with what you have identified (see Chapter 12). This is not easy – there are large amounts of information from the research to be sorted through to work out what might apply and what does not [14]. This is another purpose of the databases – not only to improve identification of relevant evidence but also to highlight the most relevant part of the evidence for different decision-making audiences.

Responding to these challenges [15], many health research bodies have endeavoured to make research easier to find by undertaking two related activities: building special collections with a browse model of searching to make research easier to find and summarising systematic reviews for easy dissemination and rapid digestion [16]. Examples of major databases are listed in Box 9.1. Such databases, combined with appropriate taxonomic structures, provide a quick way to find evidence and are often structured in a way that helps people think their way through to the intervention evidence or provide gateways to other resources. Other benefits include providing scope for easier analysis of gaps in the evidence or allowing easier comparative analysis of options.

The purpose of the specialised evidence resources varies as does the format. For example, some include full reviews; some only listings of references or reports; some summaries of reviews or summaries plus commentary. The scientific methods used to summarise reviews are also developing – a component of knowledge transfer (see Chapter 17).

Box 9.1 International databases of evidence for systems decision-making

Policy Liaison Network, Australia

www.cochrane.org.au/ebpnetwork/ is an Australian site maintained by the Australasian Cochrane Centre, funded by the Australian Department of Health and Ageing, and supporting collaboration between policy makers and researchers. The database houses summaries prepared in a standard format, including research gaps, in national health priority areas.

Health Systems Evidence, Canada

www.healthsystemsevidence.org is a Canadian website, which describes its role as a 'continuously updated repository of syntheses of research evidence about governance, financial and delivery arrangements within health systems, and about implementation strategies that can support change in health systems'. It is a collaboration of people at McMaster University, the Canadian Cochrane Centre and the Rx for Change database, established by the Canadian Agency for Drugs and Technologies in Health (CADTH) (see below). Evidence resources are organised by health systems topics and the collection includes policy briefs in addition to systematic reviews, overviews and other resources.

RX for Change, Canada

www.cadth.ca/index.php/en/compus/optimal-ther-resources/interventions is the entry point for the Rx for Change database, which provides synthesised summaries of key findings from systematic reviews about the effects of interventions targeting professionals, healthcare organisations, policy makers and consumers to improve medicines prescribing and use. It is maintained by the CADTH, through its Canadian Optimal Medication Prescribing and Utilization Service, in collaboration with the Cochrane Effective Practice and Organisation of Care (EPOC), and the Cochrane Consumers and Communication Review Group.

NHS Centre for Reviews and Dissemination, the United Kingdom

www.york.ac.uk/inst/crd/ is the York University, National Institute of Health Research, site for several major databases. Two relevant to systems decision-making are the *NHS Economic Evaluation Database* (NHS EED), containing abstracts of health economics papers and quality assessed economic evaluations; and the *Health Technology Assessment* (HTA) database, containing details of completed and ongoing health technology assessments from around the world.

> **National Library of Medicine, National Institutes of Health, USA**
> http://www.nlm.nih.gov/hsrph.html is an American site for health services research and public health programmes, including health services research databases and health technology assessments. Links to evidence reports cover both reviews of evidence for clinical treatments and evidence for improving the delivery and communication of care.

Investment needed to develop and maintain databases is substantial. As such they promote the collaborative philosophy that has allowed government agencies, researchers, clinicians and increasingly consumer organisations to work together to gather the evidence required to make informed healthcare decisions [17].

What kinds of interventions would improve health experiences?

The secondary analysis described in this chapter was conducted to identify all systematic reviews relevant to promoting health and improving the experience of illness and treatment. This phrase covers a very broad range of strategies and settings. Evidence is not currently categorised in this way, so hand searching was undertaken. The Cochrane Database of Systematic Reviews on *The Cochrane Library*, a database with a large number of relevant reviews, was hand searched at two time points: Issue 1, 2006 and 2009, to identify the number of relevant reviews and protocols (i.e. reviews that are under way), the spread of evidence in relation to key stages or states of health, illness and treatment, and the growth in evidence over time. Searching, selection and coding were undertaken by authors DL and RR.

All reviews had to meet two criteria:

- Included trials in the review were of interventions which would affect the way people interact with or experience health or the health system.
- Interventions would require systems decision-making for implementation.

Five broad categories were developed to categorise and group the reviews. The categories are informative at a browsing level, but are somewhat arbitrary. This was because a broad and inclusive categorisation associated with health experiences was chosen to enable a coding system to be placed over the top of complex and overlapping research questions at the systematic review level. The categories, simple definitions and an illustrative Cochrane review are as follows:

1 Interventions for the prevention of a disease or problem: where interventions aim to promote health and healthy behaviours.
   - *Interactive computer-based interventions for sexual health promotion* [18]

2 Interventions for the maintenance of health for people with chronic illness: where interventions aim to enable, maintain or support health-related behaviours.

- *Culture-specific programmes for children and adults from minority groups who have asthma* [19]

3 Interventions related to screening behaviours: where interventions aim to promote informed decisions and behaviours related to screening.

- *Disclosing to parents newborn carrier status identified by routine blood spot screening* [20]

4 Interventions to prepare for treatment or an episode of care: where interventions aim or enable immediate preparation for an event or episode of care.

- *Audio recordings of consultations with doctors for parents of critically sick babies* [21]

5 Interventions to inform, promote participation or improve the responsiveness of care: where interventions aim to improve the continuity or patient centredness of care.

- *Discharge planning from hospital to home* [22]

Growth in evidence for systems decision-making

In 2009, there were a total of 510 Cochrane reviews and protocols relevant to improving health experiences, up from 323 in 2006. Figure 9.1 shows the breakdown of reviews and protocols (protocols are the published plans for reviews) for the two publication periods.

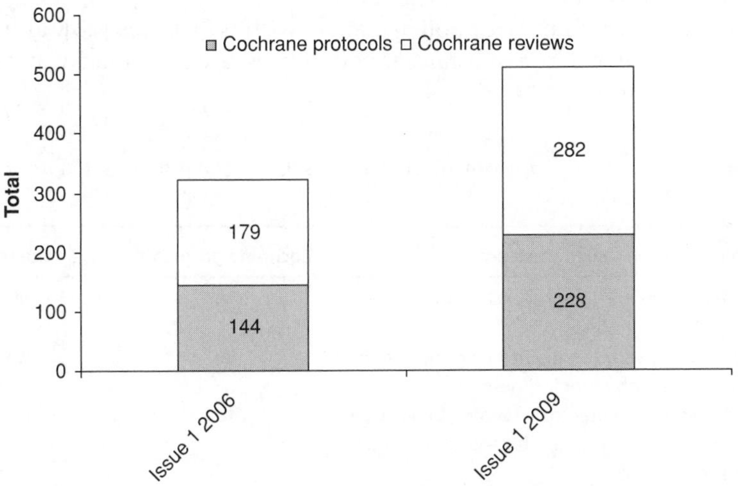

Figure 9.1 Growth in evidence of interventions to promote health and improve the experience of illness and treatment, 2006–2009.

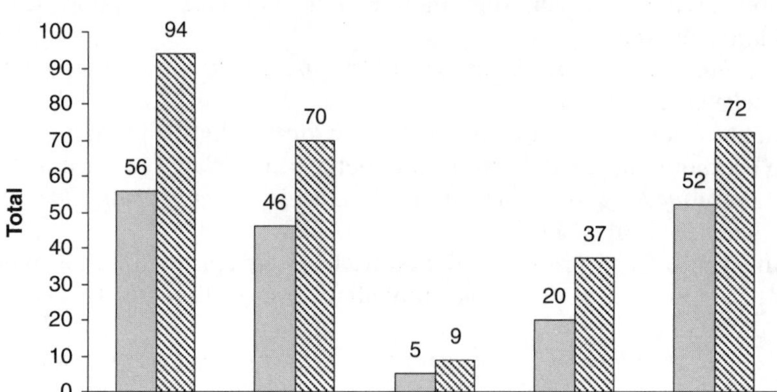

Figure 9.2 Number of Cochrane reviews by health systems category, 2006–2009.

When coded and grouped by categories, there was a wide range in reviews available for different health systems purposes (see Figure 9.2). Reviews of interventions for prevention of a disease or problem were the highest number, up from 56 to 94, no doubt reflecting a major preoccupation of governments and researchers.

Gaps in research present policy makers with difficulties [23], although Table 9.1 shows that a substantial body of research is under way across all the categories.

Table 9.1 Evidence for improving health systems, Cochrane protocols and reviews from Issue 1, 2009.

Systems decision-making categories	Cochrane protocols	Cochrane reviews
1 Interventions for the prevention of a disease or problem	70	94
2 Interventions for the maintenance of health for people with chronic illness	60	70
3 Interventions related to screening behaviours	13	9
4 Interventions to prepare for treatment or an episode of care	21	37
5 Interventions to inform, promote participation or improve the responsiveness of care	64	72

As the interest in evidence in healthcare continues to increase and the growth in the amount of research continues, expert-maintained rapid searching facilities in specialised areas will remain a valuable tool to help interested parties to locate, access and utilise relevant research.

References

1. Dawes M, Summerskill W, Glasziou P, et al. (2005) Sicily statement on evidence-based practice. *BMC Medical Education* **5**, 1.
2. Eccles MP, Armstrong D, Baker R, et al. (2009) An implementation research agenda. *Implementation Science* **4**, 18.
3. Schoen C, Osborn R, Huynh P, et al. (2005) Taking the pulse of health care systems: experiences of patients with health problems in six countries. *Health Affairs – Web Exclusive*, W5–509.
4. Forster AJ, Clark HD, Menard A, et al. (2004) Adverse events among medical patients after discharge from hospital. *Canadian Medical Association journal* **170**, 345–349.
5. Brownson RC, Fielding JE, Maylahn CM (2009) Evidence-based public health: a fundamental concept for public health practice. *Annual Review of Public Health* **30**, 175–201.
6. Victorian Quality Council (VQC) (2007) *Communicating With Consumers and Carers – Part 1 – Pilot of Evidence-Based Selection of Communication Strategies to Improve Communication Between Consumers/Carers and Health Services*. VQC, Melbourne. Available from: http://www.health.vic.gov.au/qualitycouncil/activities/consumers.htm. Accessed: 25 October 2010.
7. Victorian Quality Council (VQC) (2007) *Communicating With Consumers and Carers – Part 2 – A Guide for an Evidence-Informed Approach to Improving Communication and Participation in Health Care*. VQC, Melbourne. Available from: http://www.health.vic.gov.au/qualitycouncil/activities/consumers.htm. Accessed: 25 October 2010.
8. Clarke M (2007) The Cochrane Collaboration and systematic reviews. *British Journal of Surgery* **94**, 391–392.
9. Campbell DM, Redman S, Jorm L, Cooke M, Zwi AB, Rychetnik L (2009) Increasing the use of evidence in health policy: practice and views of policy makers and researchers. *Australia and New Zealand Health Policy* **6**, 21.
10. Green LW, Ottoson JM, Garcia C, Hiatt RA (2009) Diffusion theory and knowledge dissemination, utilization, and integration in public health. *Annual Review of Public Health* **30**, 151–174.
11. Lavis JN, Lomas J, Hamid M, Sewankambo N (2006) Assessing country-level efforts to link research to action. *Bulletin of the World Health Organization* **84**, 620–628.
12. Bidwell S (2004) Finding the evidence: resources and skills for locating information on clinical effectiveness. Evidence based medicine and healthcare. *Singapore Medical Journal* **45**, 567–572.
13. Shepperd S, Lewin S, Straus S, et al. (2009) Can we systematically review studies that evaluate complex interventions? *Public Library of Science Medicine* **6**, e1000086.
14. Cumpston M, Brennan S, Misso M, Murphy M, Green S (eds.) (2009) [O01-1] Future directions for the Cochrane Policy Liaison Initiative: a long-term knowledge

transfer and exchange partnership with the Australian Department of Health and Ageing. *17th Cochrane Colloquium*, Singapore, 11–14 October 2009.

15. Misso M, Brennan S, Green S (2006) [P092] Encouraging and supporting Australian policy makers to use Cochrane reviews – further reporting of a three year initiative. 14th Cochrane Colloquium, Dublin, 23–26 October 2006.
16. Lavis JN (2009) How can we support the use of systematic reviews in policymaking? *Public Library of Science Medicine* **6**, e1000141.
17. Volmink J, Siegfried N, Robertson K, Gülmezoglu AM (2004) Research synthesis and dissemination as a bridge to knowledge management: the Cochrane Collaboration. *Bulletin of the World Health Organization* **82**, 10.
18. Bailey JV, Murray E, Rait G, et al. (2010) Interactive computer-based interventions for sexual health promotion. *Cochrane Database of Systematic Reviews*, CD006483.
19. Bailey EJ, Cates CJ, Kruske SG, Morris PS, Brown N, Chang AB (2009) Culture-specific programs for children and adults from minority groups who have asthma. *Cochrane Database of Systematic Reviews*, CD006580.
20. Oliver S, Dezateux C, Kavanagh J, Lempert T, Stewart R (2004) Disclosing to parents newborn carrier status identified by routine blood spot screening. *Cochrane Database of Systematic Reviews*, CD003859.
21. Koh G, Budge D, Butow P, Renison B, Woodgate PG (2005) Audio recordings of consultations with doctors for parents of critically sick babies. *Cochrane Database of Systematic Reviews*, CD004502.
22. Shepperd S, McClaran J, Phillips CO, et al. (2010) Discharge planning from hospital to home. *Cochrane Database of Systematic Reviews*, CD000313.
23. Jewell CJ, Bero LA (2008) 'Developing good taste in evidence': facilitators of and hindrances to evidence-informed health policymaking in state government. *The Milbank Quarterly* **86**, 177–208.

CHAPTER 10

Looking at online health information more critically

John Kis-Rigo
Trials Search Coordinator, Cochrane Consumers and Communication Review Group, Centre for Health Communication and Participation, Australian Institute for Primary Care and Ageing, La Trobe University, Victoria, Australia

Information, health, literacy and education

When looking at matters related to a knowledgeable use of online health information by people, there is a strong temptation to use terms such as 'critical health literacy'. For some time now, an ever-growing literature has discussed, interpreted and reinterpreted the various 'literacies': health literacy, computer literacy, digital literacy, information literacy and media literacy [1, 2]. And no matter how ill-defined those may be, it is routinely claimed that their highest form is the 'critical' form.

In the information jungle, especially on the internet, users of health information should indeed be critical: trying to distinguish good advice from bad advice; learning to see paths and connections; avoiding the traps and pitfalls.

But the danger is that in adopting certain brands of 'critical literacy' we uncritically adopt their narrow ideological bases and slanted analyses when in fact people should be enabled to criticise those ideological bases and analyses too. The kind of critical sense needed is one which is perceptive enough to see through and look beyond political, ideological, academic and other 'fashions' in ideas. That critical sense is not easy to develop, either for patients or for health professionals.

Health literacy for the 'information age' needs an 'information literacy' as a central component. Information literacy has a variety of definitions and models. According to a widely used definition [3], it is a set of abilities; it means to '... recognize when information is needed and to have the ability to locate, evaluate and use effectively the needed

The Knowledgeable Patient: Communication and Participation in Health – A Cochrane Handbook, First Edition.
Edited by Sophie Hill.

information'. This definition may sound too simple – particularly in the context of other similar definitions of information literacy and the various competency standards associated with them. It is no wonder, then, that conceptions of information literacy are subject to continuing challenges and reinterpretations [4, 5].

One of the ongoing debates around the concept has been whether it is mainly generic or situated within the context of a discipline [6]. Accordingly, one major category of information literacy programmes aims at developing in students generally applicable and transferable 'information skills', whereas another approach is to incorporate it in teaching and learning within particular disciplines. Students in the health sciences are nowadays likely to be exposed to both the approaches.

The critical policy question is, how 'information literate' can people be – as future patients and partners in healthcare decision-making – when they graduate from schools, colleges or universities? What opportunities are there for them to embark on a process of lifelong learning? To what extent is a critical online literacy a focus of formal educational programs?

Lessons from general health literacy are applicable to searching online for information and these are useful for both patients and health professionals. These are 'background' considerations, which if kept in mind, will aid informed searching, reading, appraisal and use of information for personal and professional health reasons.

This is a large area of concern, and what follows is confined to pointing out a few key aspects that are often neglected.

Some neglected sides of information literacy

Where is the wisdom we have lost in knowledge?
Where is the knowledge we have lost in information?

T.S. ELIOT, *Choruses from 'The Rock'*

To be worthwhile, information literacy needs to provide support for real attempts at understanding. Many programs established at schools, colleges and universities worldwide and on the internet do not promote a deep understanding. However, key elements can be extracted from literacy definitions and standards, and lead to the following essentials:

1 recognise the need for information;
2 search reflectively;
3 evaluate, compare, analyse and synthesise the information found.

These elements are in interaction. For example, the third element often leads to a keener recognition of the need for more and better information. This, in turn, should influence how further searching is undertaken, how search processes are revised and what new insights are gained.

Although much advice is routinely offered about the details, a few vital aspects are frequently underemphasised or misinterpreted in practice. These are

- providing a realistic background for evaluation of resources;
- avoiding superficiality;
- noting the weaknesses and limitations, too, of databases;
- avoiding overreliance on information technology.

I will discuss each in turn.

Some background for realistic evaluation

It has long been standard practice to advise students to use checklists in evaluating books, chapters, articles, using such main points as scope, authority, timeliness and accuracy. This has been adapted to the evaluation of website content and articles found online. That can often be a shallow approach, with crucial difficulties going unrecognised. When it tries to be specific while still claiming to apply to widely differing subject areas, such advice becomes grossly misleading.

That is almost a routine failure in many information literacy programs. Even within the healthcare disciplines, clear *distinctions* ought to be made between essentially different categories of topics and different kinds of articles or websites. There are indicators of quality and accuracy when numerical measurement is central to an article and quite different indicators when ethical, cultural and philosophical issues are presented.

As to conventional warnings about the general unreliability of much information on the internet; or to drawing dividing lines between the uncontrolled, 'popular', media-based or commercial information on one side and scholarly–academic–official materials on the other; or to distinguishing between refereed and non-refereed publications – that kind of routine advice badly needs further, and realistic, clarification. If the stated or implied message is that non-official or non-academic publications are not reliable but government-endorsed or scholarly–academic publications are, then the advice becomes simplistic and misleading.

To develop a critical mind, students ought to be alerted to the following considerations instead (among others):

- It is indeed important to be aware that most websites should be used with considerable caution. It is a crucial point, for example, that the mass media is full of distortions, including its reporting on health-related issues. *But* it should be added that many scholarly journals – online or in print – are not free of misleading statements and argumentation either in more subtle ways. Materials included in most databases (or web-based collections of documents) – even if academic – are widely different in quality and reliability, ranging from the excellent to the misleading [7]. The expert or academic status of an author does not necessarily guarantee accuracy and reliability – even in peer-reviewed material. One example: the recognised excellence of an eminent scientist in specialised research does not make that scientist a reliable authority on philosophical or ethical issues as well.

- A recognition that while most of the content of government or professional association websites can be accurate, *some of the content can still be dubious or misleading* should be part of the critical sense to be developed. Commercial influences, e.g. those exerted by pharmaceutical companies [8, 9], are not necessarily absent from such official sites either. (And sometimes, subjective as it may be, an informal internet forum for patients' views contains candid information on the side effects of a medication or procedure not readily available from the more official sites – or from most practitioners.)

Extending the exercise of caution to official, government or professional association-endorsed websites is all the more warranted because it is there that deceptive biases are most difficult to spot. Smoothly blended with quality health information, materials on controversial topics can be easily made to look unbiased and objective, even when they make use of officially endorsed, but dubious, ideologies.

- There can be essential *limitations* in methods, measurements; in *particular kinds* of studies as well as within individual studies; in applicability of conclusions, etc. Even systematic reviews based on high-quality randomised-controlled trials have their natural limitations, and can sometimes have significant weaknesses and ambiguities: e.g. in not taking seriously enough the kind of harm, or adverse effects of a healthcare intervention, that are not usually measured by controlled trials [10].

Sometimes the underlying *assumptions* are even more important to note. What philosophical or ethical principles is a study – its description of a background, discussion, analysis and conclusions – based on? Is the assumption behind a healthcare intervention, or behind a review of interventions, based on truly universal values or only on sectional, e.g. Western liberal individualist, ideologies? Websites that advertise their advice as evidence-based may at times be only selectively evidence based – and partly based on ideological assumptions, often unstated.

- Is the content of a study or webpage genuinely insightful, perceptive, reflecting what is most *essential* about the issue it deals with? This can often be different from staying within the most fashionable or most heavily funded or promoted approaches at any given time.

To highlight such background considerations would be especially important for students coming from non-Western environments to study at Western institutions. But they are needed for others, too.

Avoiding superficiality

Information literacy advice ought to encourage a genuine search for insightful, in-depth understanding – not a 'critical' superficiality. True, superficiality in searching and evaluating is not something new or confined to web-based information. But there are some special dangers in the newer media.

On one side we have no shortage of futuristic predictions about how empowered and knowledgeable people will become as a result of constant exposure to the internet and to the even more amazing communication technologies to emerge in the future. The best among the enthusiasts tend to acknowledge quite a few serious dangers though, such as alienation, anxiety, erosion of privacy and professional responsibility, and more [11]. And to round out the picture, other keen observers speak in this context of the possible rise of 'the dumbest generation' [12].

Many people, before getting to scholarly online resources, have already acquired habits of internet and other electronic media use that may have lessened their capacity to read and think carefully. The kind of messages they got from the new media encouraged – despite all the surface 'interactivity' sometimes involved – unreflective, or shallowly reflective, consumption. The messages come thick and fast, with lots of noise. The use of logic and gaining of insights usually needs more time and silence.

When faced with the need to explore scholarly online resources and databases in earnest, many of us are ill-prepared to use them as carefully as they should be used.

Noting not only the strengths but also the weaknesses and limitations of databases

The many healthcare-related databases provide access, through the internet, to a huge amount of information, including scholarly articles – and that in itself is their main strength. But they have limitations and weaknesses, too, even apart from the fact that most are fee based and freely available to most people only through educational institutions and the like.

Database producers and vendors are naturally unwilling to advertise the weaknesses of their products. Librarians, too, are often more reticent than they should be about these. When students select databases to search from lists on their institution's library website, they can read the brief database descriptions, but these will not call special attention to any weaknesses.

In fact there are many weaknesses, some of which are in the following areas:

- range of journals covered;
- extent of international coverage;
- design, clarity and *consistent* application of the system of subject headings (also called keywords, or subjects) which should indicate what kind of topics the article is about;
- inclusion and quality of abstracts;
- clarity and user-friendliness of search mechanism.

Taking these weaknesses and limitations of databases into account enhances their proper use.

Avoiding overreliance on information technology

A much-needed piece of advice rarely given explicitly is to use the various features of information technology strictly as *tools* – not as guides or oracles. Yet an unwillingness to learn some simple rules of how the search mechanism of a database should be used is common, not only among students. Many people seem to think they can just leave it to the 'technology' to deliver the results. Disappointingly, one can find traces of this attitude reflected even in search strategies for some systematic reviews published in quality medical journals [13]. See Box 10.1 for a description of how database searching language and information technology must be utilised together to effectively search a database.

Box 10.1 Language and information technology – a brief example

To search a database for articles on a topic intelligently is a matter of language, understanding and using information technology as a tool. It helps if we have a realistic understanding, first, of how records of articles are produced for a database. Then, it is a matter of how we make use of that insight in our own use of language for searching.

The most important parts of records for searching on a topic are:

(a) The title of the article and the abstract or summary: it is here that the particular words and phrases referring to the topic of the article can be found embedded in the text.

(b) The assigned keywords or subject headings: these are usually taken from a 'controlled vocabulary' – a structured list of 'standard' words and phrases for topics in a particular database.

On the production side, people employed to assign subject headings to database records in order to describe the topics each article deals with need to understand an article, its meaning and what it is really about. When they do not understand it well enough, they cannot assign the most appropriately descriptive subject headings, making it that much more difficult for the searcher to find the record of the article. The process of assigning subject headings can be assisted by the use of advanced IT – text mining or other programs – but if such programs are blindly followed and human understanding is not used in a critical way to have the final say, then the end result is likely to be poor.

Searchers of a database, in turn, must understand, therefore, that a thorough search cannot depend on the use of the assigned subject headings alone. In their search they must also include search words and phrases that they anticipate to be embedded in the titles or the abstracts of the articles they are looking for.

For example, to find articles on the use of email (in various areas of healthcare), part of the search should make use of the relevant subject heading for email.

electronic mail/	[In the MEDLINE database]
email/	[In the EMBASE database]
computer-mediated communication/	[In the PsycINFO database]

But the wonder of human language, the variety of expressions with similar meanings and the richness in shades of meaning individual words and phrases may have, must also be kept in mind. That richness and variety had been available to the people who wrote the title and abstract of an article.

So a search strategy in MEDLINE (Ovid) could possibly begin as follows:

1 electronic mail/

2 (electronic mail* or email* or e-mail* or web mail* or webmail* or internet mail* or mailing list* or discussion list* or listserv*).tw.

3 ((patient or health or information or web or internet) adj portal*).tw.

4 (e-communication* or e-consult* or e-visit* or e-referral*).tw.

In this search strategy:

Line 1 is a subject heading, and picks up all articles indexed to the heading of electronic mail.

Line 2 uses an * for a truncation to pick up all spellings of the term.

Line 3 uses 'adj' to enable you to identify articles where terms are adjacent to each other in the title or abstract; e.g. *patient* is adjacent to *portal*.

Line 4 picks up different text words.

The suffix '.tw' is an instruction to pick up text words in the title or abstract.

The operator 'or' combines all the articles retrieved.

Information retrieval programs for databases will be continually developed and refined, so the example above may soon be outdated. But even the most advanced search mechanisms of the future will need to be used by the human searcher intelligently and critically – whatever the appearances and invitations to the contrary.

More generally, some computing professionals, psychologists, marketers, instructors, etc., mislead people about what can be expected from computers. The confusion will only get worse in future as computers and programs become ever more sophisticated and impressive. This will allow false impressions to be created in more plausible ways.

Writing perceptively on a central issue, human–computer interface design, Shneiderman and Plaisant [11] criticise attempts at creating anthropomorphic user interfaces. (This can take the form of presenting computers as human agents, using 'I' when the computer responds to human commands and similar devices.)

> The suggestion that computers can think, know or understand may give users an erroneous model of how computers work and what the machines' capacities are. Ultimately, the deception becomes apparent, and users may feel poorly treated.

The blurring of distinctions between human and computer; the muddying of the waters about what *understanding* really means; the transfer of even those decisions that should be genuinely human to information technology and its controllers – these can easily lead to various forms of dehumanisation and subtle manipulation.

Conclusion: a dose of realism for the future

A genuinely knowledgeable patient would need to pay attention to all the general areas outlined above, and of course a lot more. Even information about 'ordinary' health issues needs a critical sense to evaluate. In addition, there will be an increasing number of complex issues related to health, but also related to political, philosophical, ethical, cultural and other controversies. And naturally, the *specifics* of health information literacy would still need to be built up against the general background.

But if advice on key aspects of information literacy is frequently flawed, what can be expected of the ability of future patients to examine health-related information analytically and insightfully? The answer to that question would itself need to be honest, realistic and critical, not dismissive of the formidable difficulties reported in the literature. And it cannot apply in a vacuum either; what many see as a general crisis in education must also be kept in mind, along with the 'digital divide' and other deep-seated social and cultural problems worldwide.

In *After Autonomy* [14] and other work, Schneider has argued – in a different, but related, context – that the ideal of the currently dominant, Western, autonomy-centred bioethics – the fully well-informed, autonomous patient as the norm – is a mirage. In a wide-ranging discussion, referring to extensive evidence, one key aspect of the problem he notes is:

> Even if patients receive information and understand it, they cannot make good decisions unless they analyse it acutely. Here too the evidence is discouraging.

And depending on more or better education for a *genuinely* adequate remedy, Schneider goes on to argue, is illusory – one reason being that '... teaching and learning are much harder than bioethicists think'.

Another reason, it might be added, is that many who would do the teaching make less than reliable guides. The kind of teaching and learning in question here, again, is one that develops genuine perceptiveness, critical insights and respect for truth in depth.

While there is a need for an education that will actually help, rather than mislead, people in those areas, there is also a need to recognise the limitations of any improved programs. These will still lead to real patients with limitations in knowledge living in real society and not to the masses of autonomous individuals of ideological fantasy.

Recognising such limitations will enable more genuine participation, because it will rest on more realistic assumptions. In the longer term, both patients and health professionals will need to try to become better prepared to share in making good and responsible decisions.

References

1. Green J, Lo Bianco J, Wyn J (2007) Discourses in interaction: the intersection of literacy and health research internationally. *Literacy and Numeracy Studies* **15**, 19–37.
2. Nutbeam D (2008) The evolving concept of health literacy. *Social Science & Medicine* **67**, 2072–2078.
3. Association of College and Research Libraries (2000) *Information Literacy Competency Standards for Higher Education*. Association of College and Research Libraries, Chicago.
4. Lloyd A, Williamson K (2008) Towards an understanding of information literacy in context: implications for research. *Journal of Librarianship and Information Science* **40**, 3–12.
5. Partridge H, Bruce C, Tilley C (2008) Community information literacy: developing an Australian research agenda. *Libri: International Journal of Libraries and Information Services* **58**, 110–122.
6. Lupton M (2008) Evidence, argument and responsibility: first year students' experiences of information literacy when researching an essay. *Higher Education Research and Development* **27**, 399–414.
7. Vlassov V, Groves T (2010) The role of Cochrane Review authors in exposing research misconduct [editorial]. *The Cochrane Library*. Available from: http://www.thecochranelibrary.com/details/editorial/886689/The-role-of-Cochrane-Review-authors-in-exposing-research-and-publication-miscond.html#_16_. Accessed: 20 December 2010.
8. Angell M (2005) *The Truth About Drug Companies*. Scribe Publications, Victoria.
9. Moynihan R (2010) *Sex Lies and Pharmaceuticals*. Allen and Unwin, New South Wales.
10. Higgins J, Green S (eds.) (2009) *Cochrane Handbook for Systematic Reviews of Interventions Version 5.0.2*, Chapter 14. Available from: www.cochrane-handbook.org. Accessed: 14 April 2010.
11. Shneiderman B, Plaisant C (2005) *Designing the User Interface: Strategies for Effective Human-Computer Interaction,* 4th ed. Pearson/Addison Wesley, Boston.

12. Bauerlein M (2008) *The Dumbest Generation: How the Digital Age Stupefies Young Americans and Jeopardizes Our Future*. Jeremy P. Tarcher/Penguin, New York.
13. Lowe D, Ryan R, Santesso N, Hill S (2010) Development of a taxonomy of interventions to organise the evidence on consumers' medicines use. *Patient Education and Counseling,* DOI: 10.1016/j.pec.2010.1009.1024.
14. Schneider C (2006) After autonomy. *Wake Forest Law Review* **41**, 411–444.

CHAPTER 11
Learning to communicate

Megan Prictor[1], *Simon Lewin*[2], *Brian McKinstry*[3] *and Jessica Kaufman*[4]

[1]Managing Editor, Cochrane Consumers and Communication Review Group, Centre for Health Communication and Participation, Australian Institute for Primary Care and Ageing, La Trobe University, Victoria, Australia

[2]Senior Researcher, Preventive and International Care Unit, Norwegian Knowledge Centre for the Health Services, Oslo, Norway; Health Systems Research Unit, Medical Research Council of South Africa, Cape Town, South Africa

[3]Reader in Primary Care Research, Centre for Population Health Sciences, University of Edinburgh, Edinburgh, Scotland, United Kingdom

[4]Research Officer, Cochrane Consumers and Communication Review Group, Centre for Health Communication and Participation, Australian Institute for Primary Care and Ageing, La Trobe University, Bundoora, Victoria, Australia

Introduction

This chapter is about the current state of evidence and the future research agenda for educational interventions directed to health professionals and consumers to improve their ability to communicate with one another.

Interaction between healthcare providers and consumers is a key element of healthcare quality. Successful communication can positively influence patient outcomes such as treatment adherence, satisfaction with care, health status and pain management [1,2]. In contrast, poor communication is a major factor in complaints by patients [3], as well as in medical litigation [4]. Communication problems may also give rise to harmful psychological and emotional outcomes for both health professionals and patients, including anxiety, uncertainty, stress and dissatisfaction [2, 5]. Communication skills – of both health professionals and consumers – are therefore increasingly the subject of training and education interventions. In this chapter, we review and discuss the evidence for the effectiveness of training and education interventions in communication skills directed at health professionals and consumers of health services.

The Knowledgeable Patient: Communication and Participation in Health – A Cochrane Handbook, First Edition.
Edited by Sophie Hill.

Training of health professionals

Themes and context

Reflecting the shift of the physician's role from paternalistic expert to shared decision-making partner, healthcare organisations and educational facilities are increasingly emphasising the importance of improving communication with patients. Reports released by the British Medical Association (BMA) board of medical education and the American Medical Association strongly support communication skills training for doctors and other health professionals, in under- and postgraduate programmes as well as throughout their practicing careers [6–8]. In addition, the World Health Organization has incorporated communication standards into international guidance for the management of a range of health issues, including chronic diseases and tuberculosis [9].

Medical schools, responding to various influences such as increased litigation, empowerment of consumers, shifting views among providers and a changing policy environment [10], are also focusing on developing communication skills and a patient-centred approach amongst students [11]. Makoul says that the 'idea of communication as a *bedside manner* or *history taking* has given way to a reconceptualization of communication as a measurable clinical skill' [12].

Internationally, methods such as lectures, discussion, direct or video observation, role-play and practice with simulated and real patients are utilised to teach communication skills. In many medical schools, such training is a fundamental part of the undergraduate curriculum [10]. For example, a consensus statement in 2008 from all 33 UK medical schools identified key recommended curriculum content in this area [13]. The Australian Medical Council standards for basic medical education also identify communication skills as a core attribute of medical graduates [14]. In the United States, teaching and assessment of communication skills is required to obtain a medical license, although Makoul notes that there is no stipulation as to when, how or how much training must be provided [12].

Communication training in medical schools is not only undertaken in countries with well-funded medical programmes. Doctors in low- and middle-income countries face unique communication challenges, such as addressing the stigma of diseases such as HIV. Increasingly, medical education bodies in these countries are recognising the importance of good communication and implementing training programmes [15, 16].

Communication education is not limited to doctors, though the research evidence regarding the effectiveness of interventions focuses heavily on doctor training. Nursing and allied health programmes also teach and evaluate communication skills. For instance, the Nursing and Midwifery Council in the United Kingdom has specified that for registration, nurses must achieve proficiency in 'engaging in, developing and disengaging from therapeutic relationships through the use of appropriate communication and interpersonal skills' [17]. The core competency standards of the Australian Nursing and Midwifery Council require that an Australian-registered nurse 'communicates effectively with individuals/groups to facilitate provision of care' [18].

Evidence

Because effective communication is important in improving the quality of healthcare delivery as well as health outcomes, there is a need to identify ways of training and supporting healthcare professionals to communicate effectively. There is wide variation in the scope of these interventions, including who provides the intervention, what is provided, when, where, for how long, how 'intensely' and with what specific purpose. In an attempt to identify what works best, researchers have evaluated communication training for health professionals and consumers using reliable study designs such as randomised trials. These trials have been assembled and assessed in a number of systematic reviews, including some Cochrane reviews, in order to provide a clear evidence base to inform policy, practice and further research. The key features and findings of several reviews of interventions directed towards health professionals are outlined in Table 11.1.

Training of consumers

Themes and context

Training doctors to communicate more effectively cannot 'solve' the communication 'problem' on its own. Patients are also participants in communication exchange; to improve outcomes, training must be directed to consumers as well as health professionals. One review notes that patients typically express their concerns and symptoms to doctors only indirectly [22], while another reports that 'in practice patients often contribute little to the consultation apart from answering direct questions' [23]. To some degree, this phenomenon may be the result of ineffective communication by doctors, but consumer-directed training can help patients participate more actively. Some research suggests that more involved patients may have better health outcomes, such as reduced anxiety [23], although this is not yet well established. Other reviews indicate that interventions that attempt to help patients address their information needs within consultations, or to involve patients in their healthcare, do not necessarily result in better outcomes compared with usual approaches or no training [24, 25].

Methods for helping patients improve their interactions with healthcare providers (what Douglas Post has called 'the other half of the whole') have thus been explored. Researchers have tested diverse patient training interventions such as asking patients to consider their information needs and write down any questions before their consultation [24], and

Table 11.1 Description of reviews of interventions directed to the *health professional* to improve communication.

Author, year	Review objective	Features of review	Outcomes measured	Review findings
Moore et al. 2004 [2] (Cochrane review)	'To assess whether communication skills training is effective in changing health professionals' behaviour in cancer care with regard to communication/ interaction with patients'	*Types of studies*: RCTs and CBAs *Number of studies included*: 3 (all RCTs) *Participants*: healthcare professionals *Setting*: cancer care hospitals, hospices and ambulatory care settings *Interventions*: any form of communication skills training compared with other training or with no intervention	• Changes in behaviour or skills	'There is some evidence to suggest labour-intensive communications skills training can have a beneficial effect on behaviour change in professionals working with cancer patients'. However, 'it is not known whether the improvements in communication skills are of a sufficient level to be apparent to patients'
Gysels et al. 2004 [5]	'To assess the effectiveness of different communication skills training courses for health professionals in cancer care'	*Types of studies*: RCTs, CBAs, ITS *Number of studies included*: 16 *Participants*: undergraduate medical or nursing students or health professionals with experience in caring for cancer patients *Setting:* cancer care settings and undergraduate programmes *Interventions:* 'interventions focusing on basic skills as well as on attitudes with the aim of improving communication'	• Communication skills	'All the interventions demonstrated modest improvements . . . and one found deterioration in the outcomes measured'. The authors conclude that 'communication training improves basic communication skills. Positive attitudes and beliefs are needed to maintain skills over time in clinical practice and to effectively handle emotional situations'

Parry 2008 [19]	'To systematically review direct evidence about effects of interventions to improve communication performance amongst allied health professionals'; and 'to summarise indirect evidence [from other systematic reviews] pertinent to design, delivery, effects, and evaluation of such interventions'	**Direct evidence review** (review of primary studies): *Types of studies*: any *Number of studies included*: 5 *Participants*: healthcare workers including allied health professionals *Setting:* clinical and rehabilitation settings *Interventions*: 'training interventions which included a substantial or sole focus on communication skills' and where 'some form of qualitative and/or quantitative evaluation of effects was reported' For the **indirect evidence review** (summary of existing reviews), the author sought evidence from other systematic reviews 'summarising findings and arguments about: effects, recipients, modalities, content, length, and evaluation of training'. 9 reviews (2 Cochrane, 7 non-Cochrane) were included	• Interpersonal skills • Patient satisfaction • Quality of care	'There is some evidence that some communication skills training interventions can have positive effects on trainees' behaviours, quality of care, and patient satisfaction. Practical participatory modalities seem more likely to be effective' 'More empirical and conceptual understandings about AHPs' [allied health professionals'] communication practices are required so as to improve the design, delivery and subsequent evaluation of communication training amongst these important healthcare workers'
Dwamena et al. (in press) [20] (Cochrane review)	'To assess the effects of interventions for healthcare providers that aim to promote patient-centred approaches in clinical consultations'	*Types of studies:* RCTs *Number of studies included:* 41 *Participants:* healthcare providers, including providers in training *Setting:* clinical consultations in any setting (e.g. hospital in- and outpatient departments and family practice) *Interventions:* interventions that intended to promote patient-centred care within clinical consultations	• Consultation process • Patient health status • Patient satisfaction • Healthcare behaviours	Training in patient centredness for providers may result in moderate improvements in communication with patients and enable clarification of patients' concerns in consultations. However, this training rarely shows measurable effects on patient health status or satisfaction unless combined with additional interventions directed at patients and providers. It is not clear whether training in patient centredness has an impact on healthcare behaviours

(*Continued*)

Table 11.1 *(Continued)*

Author, year	Review objective	Features of review	Outcomes measured	Review findings
Légaré et al. 2010 [21] (Cochrane review)	'To determine the effectiveness of interventions to improve healthcare professionals' adoption of SDM [shared decision-making]'	*Types of studies:* RCTs, controlled clinical trials, CBAs, ITS *Number of studies included:* 5 (RCTs) *Participants:* physicians or nurses *Setting:* primary clinical care or specialised care settings *Interventions:* 'intervention[s] designed to increase healthcare professionals' adoption of SDM, defined as a process by which a healthcare choice is made jointly by the practitioner and the patient'	• Healthcare professionals' adoption of SDM • SDM as reported by the patient • Patient health outcomes • Patient and practitioner process outcomes • Practitioners' knowledge, attitudes or satisfaction with the consultation	Only two of the five included RCTs found a statistically significant effect of the intervention on healthcare professionals' adoption of SDM 'Training healthcare professionals may be important, as may the implementation of patient-mediated interventions such as decision aids. However, given the paucity of the evidence, those motivated by the ethical impetus to increase SDM in clinical practice will need to weigh the costs and potential benefits of interventions designed to increase healthcare professionals' adoption of SDM'

CBAs, controlled before-and-after studies; ITS, interrupted time-series studies; RCTs, randomised controlled trials.

coaching or modelling active participation skills in the consultation [24]. Consumer organisations have also shown leadership in promoting communication skills improvement on the part of patients. In Australia, the Consumers' Health Forum (www.chf.org.au) has produced a range of fact sheets for patients on topics such as preparing for a healthcare consultation and talking with one's pharmacist (see www.chf.org.au/factsheets.php).

A new focus on patient involvement has also followed in the wake of the Institute of Medicine's landmark report on the extent of medical mistakes [26]. National healthcare quality and safety agencies have produced a range of checklists and guides for consumers promoting healthcare safety, which encourage question asking, maintaining a list of one's medications, obtaining test results and other ways of being involved actively in one's healthcare [27, 28].

Evidence

Various ways of encouraging and educating patients to take a more proactive role in the clinical encounter have been the subject of research and evaluation. Several examples of reviews directed to consumers are outlined in Table 11.2, and key findings are summarised.

Training directed to both consumers and health professionals

Themes and context

Some training interventions are directed at both clinicians and consumers, building skills for each group by encouraging them to work collaboratively. As Rao and colleagues have pointed out, reviews which focus on only one or the other side of the communication coin impede 'our ability to view the changes in communication within the context of a conversation between 2 people' [29]. This dual approach may be particularly informative when dealing with sensitive communication issues, such as the delivery of bad news (e.g. a diagnosis of HIV infection or cancer) or notification of medical errors, which are likely to engender emotional responses from both the patient and the clinician. For instance, Gallagher notes that the doctor–patient interaction is an important feature of the response to a medical error, and communication strategies should therefore consider the attitudes of both the parties concurrently rather than look at each in isolation [30]. Gallagher describes a method for integrating the experiences of patients and physicians: he combines a patients-only focus group with a physicians-only group and allows first one and then the other to talk amongst themselves about medical errors while the other group listens. At the end, the groups discuss the issue together.

Patients may also be involved in the training and education of physicians. The value of this collaboration is recognised in a recent BMA

Table 11.2 Description of reviews of interventions directed to the *consumer* to improve communication.

Author, year	Review objective	Features of review	Outcomes measured	Review findings
Harrington et al. 2004 [23]	'To examine intervention studies designed to increase patients' participation in medical consultations'	*Types of studies*: various, including randomised placebo-controlled experimental designs *Number of studies included*: 20 *Participants*: patients or volunteers simulating patients (one study) *Setting:* outpatient or primary care settings *Interventions:* interventions (written, face-to-face coaching and videotapes) designed to improve patients' communication with their doctors	• Patient satisfaction • Perceptions of control over health • Preferences for an active role in healthcare • Recall of information • Adherence to recommendations • Attendance • Clinical outcomes	'The studies considered in this review generally demonstrated that interventions directed at patients can be successful in increasing patient participation, and that, in some circumstances, this can be achieved without an increase in consultation length' 'Encouraging patient participation appeared to lead to a greater sense of control and preference for a more active role in consultations in a number of studies, although the results were less clear when considering satisfaction, knowledge, and recall'

Wetzels et al. 2004 [25] (Cochrane review)	'To assess the effects of interventions in primary medical care that improve the involvement of older patients (≥65 years) in their health care'	*Types of studies*: RCTs or quasi-RCTs *Number of studies included*: 3 *Participants*: older patients (≥65 years of age) *Setting:* home and office primary care encounters *Interventions:* written or face-to-face interventions to improve older people's involvement in their care	• Questioning or active behaviour • Patient satisfaction	'Interventions of a pre-visit booklet and a pre-visit session . . . led to more questioning behaviour and more self-reported active behaviour' However, due to the limited evidence, the authors 'cannot recommend the use of the reviewed interventions in daily practice. There should be a balance between respecting patients' autonomy and stimulating their active participation in health care. Face-to-face coaching sessions . . . may be the way forward'
Kinnersley et al. 2007 [24] (Cochrane review)	'To assess the effects on patients, clinicians and the healthcare system of interventions which are delivered before consultations, and which have been designed to help patients (and/or their representatives) address their information needs within consultations'	*Types of studies*: RCTs *Number of studies included*: 33 (all RCTs) *Participants*: patients and/or their representatives or carers before consultations *Setting:* a range of settings *Interventions:* interventions (e.g. question checklists and patient coaching) delivered 'before consultations and designed to encourage question asking and information gathering by the patient'	• Question asking • Patient participation • Patient anxiety • Knowledge • Satisfaction • Consultation length	'The interventions seem to help patients ask more questions in consultations, but do not have other clear benefits. Doctors and nurses need to continue to try to help their patients ask questions in consultations and question prompt sheets or coaching may help in some circumstances'

RCTs, randomised controlled trials.

Medical Education Subcommittee publication. According to the paper, patient contact during physician training gives students the opportunity to 'learn and to develop their professional skills, attitudes and identity'. Patients benefit both directly and indirectly 'by increasing their own knowledge, and ... through improved training of the medical workforce' [31].

Evidence

Promoting the involvement and communication skills of patients and doctors is no longer seen as simply 'good to do', but rather as crucial to efforts to improve health systems and outcomes. Table 11.3 features reviews of interventions directed to both patients and health professionals and summarises their key findings.

Discussion and conclusions

Gaps in the evidence

Training to improve communication is an evolving field of research and practice, so it is not surprising that when we look for evidence about methods of improving the communication skills of health professionals or consumers, results are mixed and there are gaps in the available information. Gaps may be a consequence of the structure and focus of existing primary studies or of the scope of systematic reviews. We have organised the discussion of evidence gaps according to the populations covered by studies, the intervention evaluated, the comparisons made and the outcomes measured.

Population

Gaps in a study population can produce skewed results, or results that are not applicable to significant groups of healthcare consumers. If the sampled group towards which an intervention is directed is less heterogeneous (i.e. mixed) than the larger population from which it is drawn, the results of a study may not be generalisable to this wider population. For example, several Cochrane reviews suggest that conducting trials with doctors who are already interested in improving their communication skills may result in very positive outcomes that are unlikely to be achieved among the population of doctors as a whole [2, 32]. Conversely, it could be that interested doctors are already relatively good communicators, and therefore, a noticeable improvement in their communication skills may be unlikely. Future trials should include populations of health professionals with no expressed interest in communication, through directing interventions at all professionals in a geographic area or organisation.

Studies also tend to focus on the most accessible populations, which leads to gaps in evidence for groups at either end of the age spectrum. Children and adults over 65 years of age are both groups that are

Table 11.3 Description of reviews of interventions directed to the *consumer and health professional* to improve communication.

Author, year	Review objective	Features of review	Outcomes measured	Review findings
McKinstry et al. 2006 [32] (Cochrane review)	'To assess the effects of interventions intended to improve a patient's trust in the doctor or a group of doctors'	*Types of studies*: RCTs, quasi-RCTs, CBAs, ITS *Number of studies included*: 3 (all RCTs) *Participants*: doctors, healthcare consumers and their relatives *Setting:* North American primary care *Interventions:* 'any intervention (for example informative, educational, behavioural, organisational) directed at doctors or patients (or carers) that was intended to influence patients' trust in their doctors'	• Trust	'Overall there remains insufficient evidence to conclude that any intervention may increase or decrease trust in doctors. Further trials are required to explore the impact of policy changes, guidelines and specific doctors' training on patients' trust'
Rao et al. 2007 [29]	'To synthesize the findings of studies examining interventions to enhance the communication behaviors of physicians and patients during outpatient encounters'	*Types of studies*: RCTs *Number of studies included*: 36 *Participants*: physicians and patients *Setting:* primary care clinics and medical specialty settings *Interventions:* communication interventions (e.g. information, feedback, modelling, practice) designed to improve the communication behaviours of physicians and patients	• Verbal communication behaviours	'In general, the interventions resulted in enhanced communication behaviors among physicians. Compared with controls, intervention physicians were more likely to receive higher global ratings of their communication style and to exhibit specific patient-centered communication behaviors. Similar, modest effects occurred with patient interventions. Intervention patients obtained more information per question and exhibited greater involvement during the visit than controls'

(*Continued*)

Table 11.3 (*Continued*)

Author, year	Review objective	Features of review	Outcomes measured	Review findings
Watson and McKinstry 2009 [33]	'To carry out a systematic review of intervention trials designed to enhance recall of medical information'	*Types of studies*: RCTs, controlled trials, randomised trials *Number of studies included*: 34 *Participants*: healthcare professionals and patients engaged in interaction *Setting:* clinical setting *Interventions:* any 'preconceived intervention (e.g. written material, audio recordings, specific presentation styles, etc.) specifically designed to test its comparative effect on recall/knowledge of clinical instruction/consultation/counselling advice'	• Recall performance	'While written and tape-recorded instructions appear to improve recall in most situations . . . further research is required in clinical settings to determine if cognitive interventions based on a more over-arching psychological model of recall are effective'

CBAs, controlled before-and-after studies; ITS, interrupted time-series studies; RCTs, randomised controlled trials.

largely absent from existing reviews on communication skills, a paradox given that these age groups are frequent consumers of health services. For example, Kinnersley and colleagues' extensive review [24] of pre-consultation preparation identified only one study [34] addressing communication with parents of a paediatric population. Reviews about communication with children [35, 36] identified studies that focus primarily on information provision, support and education, but not directly on enhancing the health-related communication skills of the child as a patient, the parents or siblings, or the health professionals involved. With regard to older adults, Wetzels and colleagues note that 'despite abundant literature on involvement, there are few trials focussed solely on older populations'. The review authors identified only three studies of older adults, even though people in this group are the main consumers of healthcare [25].

There is also a dearth of studies focusing on healthcare professionals other than doctors, such as nurses and allied professionals. Given the importance of these cadres in delivering healthcare across many settings, particularly in primary care, studies are needed to explore the effects of interventions to improve communication between these healthcare providers and patients, as well as between teams of professionals and patients.

When considering the populations included in these studies, setting is a potentially overlooked feature. Most of the studies included in these reviews were conducted in North America, Europe or Australia. There appears to be few studies from low- and middle-income countries on interventions to improve communication within consultations, and this raises questions about the applicability of the available evidence to such settings. Differences in cultures, on-the-ground realities and constraints and in health systems arrangements between high- and low-income settings may substantially alter the feasibility and acceptability of such interventions, or may mean that these do not have the same effects [37].

Interventions

A number of communication skills interventions and topics have not yet been reviewed systematically. One of these is the role of carers, including family members, in the consultation process – a facet of communication which is often absent from discussion and research in the field. Recent reviews highlight a new focus on carer issues [38, 39]; however, to date there is no Cochrane review specifically assessing communication interventions directed at carers who participate in consultations or examining the training of health professionals to communicate more effectively with them.

Another communication area with limited research is the training of health professionals to use new forms of consultation – particularly telephone-based consultations. In many countries, telephonic conversation has become the standard form of first consultation out of hours, and it increasingly is forming a significant proportion of daytime consultations too [40]. A Cochrane review on the effects of telephone-based consultation on patient satisfaction and health outcomes found studies suggesting that the service is safe and may reduce general practitioner (GP) visits. However, the review did not specifically address the communication challenges that may be unique to telephone-based consultation or to physician training in this form of communication [41].

Comparisons

Some reviews suggested that further research into communication training should look at comparisons between interventions, rather than examine individual approaches in isolation [2]. When deciding between using a training intervention or doing nothing, it may be logical to compare the results of the intervention with those of a control group. However, developing and determining the most effective intervention for a given setting requires a direct comparison of different approaches. As the importance of improving communication through interventions becomes more recognised, studies will focus on the fine-tuning of interventions and this kind of comparison will become increasingly common.

Outcomes

There are gaps in the outcomes measured by trialists, with the bulk of available data relating to patient satisfaction and the number (but not the quality) of questions asked of doctors. Review authors have identified the need for trials to assess a much broader range of outcomes, including objective measures of healthcare behaviours and health status (e.g. blood pressure and adherence to treatment). However, it may be optimistic to expect significant effects on these outcomes given the nature, scope and timing of many communication interventions. These interventions may be quite small scale, in relation to the overall history of communication between the professional and the patient regarding a particular health issue. They may also influence proximal outcomes, such as knowledge or understanding, but their overall effects may be difficult to isolate among the many other factors that influence more distal outcomes such as health status. Ideally, with a broader range of measured outcomes in studies, review authors would be better able to identify the areas in which the interventions have produced significant results. There is also a need to measure outcomes at longer post-intervention intervals to determine whether intervention effects are sustained over time.

There are a myriad different outcomes, as well as outcome assessment tools, used in communication intervention trials. For many outcome areas, such as 'patient centredness', there is still no widely accepted 'gold-standard' measure that can be used across studies to make the results more comparable. Taxonomies of outcomes may help us to better understand the relations between these different measures. The Cochrane Consumers and Communication Review Group's taxonomy of outcomes is a useful tool for grouping the outcomes used in these kinds of studies (www.latrobe.edu.au/chcp/assets/downloads/Outcomes.pdf).

The language used to discuss outcomes can also have a significant impact on comparative analysis between studies (see Chapter 4). For instance, there is an overlap between some of the constructs that form the focus of several of the systematic reviews in this field, including 'trust', 'patient-centred care' and 'shared decision-making'. It is not always clear how these outcomes differ and the implications of these differences for implementing interventions intended to enhance them. Standardising language through tools like the taxonomy of outcomes is one solution to improving our conceptual understanding of the links between these communication constructs and the effects of interventions designed to promote them [42].

Putting evidence into practice

Most of the reviews suggest that interventions to improve communication between clinicians and patients have only modest benefits on consultation processes and patient satisfaction. This may suggest that these interventions are not worth the effort required to implement them, but there are a number of possible reasons for the modest effects found. One factor that may have influenced the results is that many of the interventions were fairly small in scale and may not have been able to achieve a measurable impact on outcomes. Additionally, tools to assess outcomes such as patient satisfaction may not be able to detect subtle changes in these outcomes following a consultation. Finally, consultations are complex interactions and often part of a long-standing relationship between the clinician and the patient. Cross-sectional assessments of outcomes may not capture adequately the nature of these ongoing relationships.

Notwithstanding the gaps identified above, and the lack of clear and consistent messages across the existing reviews, we can still put the research evidence to good use. Where we have confidence in the findings of a systematic review, and these indicate clear benefits and few harms (e.g. improved patient satisfaction from interventions to promote patient-centred care in the clinical consultation), decision-makers may want to consider implementing such interventions. There may in fact be an ethical imperative to implement interventions that result in increased patient satisfaction – even if these do not produce improved health outcomes – as it is generally accepted that patients have a right to adequate communication with their clinician. Where the research has promising findings, but there is insufficient evidence to be confident about its effects, consideration should be given to implementing the intervention(s) in the context of evaluation [43].

Conclusion

Existing systematic reviews may help to bring patient-centred communication to the fore in discussions of healthcare quality by indicating that communication interventions can, and should, be informed by high-quality evidence. Involving patients, clinicians and other stakeholders in discussions regarding which interventions to implement may help to address questions of the applicability of the existing body of evidence to a particular setting.

References

1. van Nuland M, Hannes K, Aertgeerts B, Goedhuys J (2005) Educational interventions for improving the communication skills of general practice trainees in the clinical consultation (Protocol). *Cochrane Database of Systematic Reviews*, CD005559.
2. Moore PM, Wilkinson SSM, Rivera Mercado S (2004) Communication skills training for health care professionals working with cancer patients, their families and/or carers. *Cochrane Database of Systematic Reviews*, CD003751.
3. Wofford MM, Wofford JL, Bothra J, Kendrick SB, Smith A, Lichstein PR (2004) Patient complaints about physician behaviors: a qualitative study. *Academic Medicine* **79**, 134–138.
4. Levinson W, Roter DL, Mullooly JP, Dull VT, Frankel RM (1997) Physician-patient communication. The relationship with malpractice claims among primary care physicians and surgeons. *Journal of the American Medical Association* **277**, 553–559.
5. Gysels M, Richardson A, Higginson IJ (2004) Communication training for health professionals who care for patients with cancer: a systematic review of effectiveness. *Supportive Care in Cancer* **12**, 692–700.
6. British Medical Association (2004) *Communication Education Skills for Doctors: An Update*. Available from: http://uk.sitestat.com/bma/bma/s?communication.pdf&ns_type=pdf&ns_url=http://www.bma.org.uk/images/communication_tcm41-20207.pdf. Accessed: 23 March 2010.
7. American Medical Association (2007) *Initiative to Transform Medical Education: Recommendations for Change in the System of Medical Education*. Available from: http://www.ama-assn.org/ama1/pub/upload/mm/377/itme-final.pdf. Accessed: 23 March 2010.
8. American Medical Association (2006) *Improving Communication—Improving Care: An Ethical Force Program™ Consensus Report*. Available from: http://www.ama-assn.org/ama1/pub/upload/mm/369/ef_imp_comm.pdf. Accessed: 23 March 2010.
9. World Health Organization (2006) *The Stop TB Strategy: Building on and Enhancing DOTS to Meet the TB-related Millennium Development Goals*. Geneva. Available from: http://whqlibdoc.who.int/hq/2006/WHO_HTM_STB_2006.368_eng.pdf. Accessed: 28 April 2010.
10. Brown J (2008) How clinical communication has become a core part of medical education in the UK. *Medical Education* **42**, 271–278.
11. Haidet P, Kelly PA, Bentley S, et al. (2006) Not the same everywhere. Patient-centered learning environments at nine medical schools. *Journal of General Internal Medicine* **21**, 405–409.

12. Makoul G (2003) Communication skills education in medical school and beyond. *Journal of the American Medical Association* **289**, 93.
13. von Fragstein M, Silverman J, Cushing A, Quilligan S, Salisbury H, Wiskin C (2008) UK consensus statement on the content of communication curricula in undergraduate medical education. *Medical Education* **42**, 1100–1107.
14. Australian Medical Council (2009) *Assessment and Accreditation of Medical Schools: Standards and Procedures*. Available from: http://www.amc.org.au/images/Medschool/standards.pdf. Accessed: 6 January 2010.
15. Houston S, Ray S, Chitsike I, et al. (2005) Breaking the silence: an HIV-related educational intervention for medical students in Zimbabwe. *The Central African Journal of Medicine* **51**, 48–52.
16. White J, Kruger C, Snyman W (2008) Development and implementation of communication skills in dentistry: an example from South Africa. *European Journal of Dental Education* **12**, 29–34.
17. Nursing and Midwifery Council (2004) *Standards of Proficiency for Pre-registration Nursing Education*. London. Available from: http://www.nmc-uk.org/aDisplayDocument.aspx?documentID=328. Accessed: 28 April 2010.
18. Australian Nursing and Midwifery Council (2006) *National Competency Standards for the Registered Nurse*. Available from: http://www.anmc.org.au/userfiles/file/RN%20Competency%20Standards%20August%202008%20(new%20format).pdf. Accessed: 23 March 2010.
19. Parry R (2008) Are interventions to enhance communication performance in allied health professionals effective, and how should they be delivered? Direct and indirect evidence. *Patient Education and Counseling* **73**, 186–195.
20. Dwamena F, Sikorskii A, Holmes-Rovner M, et al. (In press) Interventions for providers to promote a patient-centred approach in clinical consultations. *Cochrane Database of Systematic Reviews*.
21. Légaré F, Ratté S, Stacey D, et al. (2010) Interventions for improving the adoption of shared decision making by healthcare professionals. *Cochrane Database of Systematic Reviews*, CD006732.
22. Post D, Cegala D, Miser W (2002) The other half of the whole: teaching patients to communicate with physicians. *Family Medicine* **34**, 344–352.
23. Harrington J, Noble L, Newman S (2004) Improving patients' communication with doctors: a systematic review of intervention studies. *Patient Education and Counseling* **52**, 7–16.
24. Kinnersley P, Edwards A, Hood K, et al. (2007) Interventions before consultations for helping patients address their information needs. *Cochrane Database of Systematic Reviews*, CD004565.
25. Wetzels R, Harmsen M, Van Weel C, Grol R, Wensing M (2007) Interventions for improving older patients' involvement in primary care episodes. *Cochrane Database of Systematic Reviews*, CD004273.
26. Kohn LT, Corrigan JM, Donaldson MS (eds.) (2000) *To Err Is Human: Building a Safer Health System*. National Academy Press, Washington.
27. Agency for Healthcare Research and Quality (2004) *Five Steps to Safer Health Care: Patient Fact Sheet*. US Department of Health and Human Services. Available from: http://www.ahrq.gov/consumer/5steps.htm. Accessed: 14 April 2010.
28. Australian Council for Safety and Quality in Health Care (2003) *Ten Tips for Safer Health Care*. Available from: http://www.health.gov.au/internet/safety/publishing.

nsf/Content/BE79FB82644728ABCA2571C0000330FB/$File/10tipsclnbox.pdf. Accessed: 14 April 2010.

29. Rao J, Anderson L, Inui T, Frankel R (2007) Communication interventions make a difference in conversations between physicians and patients: a systematic review of the evidence. *Medical Care* **45**, 340–349.
30. Gallagher TH, Waterman AD, Ebers AG, Fraser VJ, Levinson W (2003) Patients' and physicians' attitudes regarding the disclosure of medical errors. *Journal of the American Medical Association* **289**, 1001–1007.
31. British Medical Association (2008) *Role of the Patient in Medical Education*. Available from: http://www.bma.org.uk/images/roleofthepatient_tcm41-175953.pdf. Accessed: 23 March 2010.
32. McKinstry B, Ashcroft R, Car J, Freeman GK, Sheikh A (2006) Interventions for improving patients' trust in doctors and groups of doctors. *Cochrane Database of Systematic Reviews*, CD004134.
33. Watson PW, McKinstry B (2009) A systematic review of interventions to improve recall of medical advice in healthcare consultations. *Journal of the Royal Society of Medicine* **102**, 235–243.
34. Lewis C, Pantell R, Sharp L (1991) Increasing patient knowledge, satisfaction, and involvement: randomized trial of a communication intervention. *Pediatrics* **88**, 351–358.
35. Ranmal R, Prictor M, Scott JT (2008) Interventions for improving communication with children and adolescents about their cancer. *Cochrane Database of Systematic Reviews*, CD002969.
36. Scott JT, Prictor M, Harmsen M, et al. (2003) Interventions for improving communication with children and adolescents about a family member's cancer. *Cochrane Database of Systematic Reviews*, CD004511.
37. Lavis JN, Oxman AD, Souza NM, Lewin S, Gruen RL, Fretheim A (2009) SUPPORT Tools for evidence-informed health Policymaking (STP) 9: Assessing the applicability of the findings of a systematic review. *Health Research Policy and Systems* **7**, S9.
38. Candy B, Jones L, Williams R, Tookman A, King M (2009) Interventions for supporting informal caregivers of patients in the terminal phase of a disease (Protocol). *Cochrane Database of Systematic Reviews*, CD007617.
39. Smith J, Forster A, House A, Knapp P, Wright JJ, Young J (2008) Information provision for stroke patients and their caregivers. *Cochrane Database of Systematic Reviews*, CD001919.
40. McKinstry B, Watson P, Pinnock H, Heaney D, Sheikh A (2009) Telephone consulting in primary care: a triangulated qualitative study of patients and providers. *The British Journal of General Practice* **59**, e209–218.
41. Bunn F, Byrne G, Kendall S (2004) Telephone consultation and triage: effects on health care use and patient satisfaction. *Cochrane Database of Systematic Reviews*, CD004180.
42. Shepperd S, Lewin S, Straus S, et al. (2009) Can we systematically review studies that evaluate complex interventions? *PLoS Medicine* **6**, e1000086.
43. Oxman AD, Lavis JN, Fretheim A, Lewin S (2009) SUPPORT Tools for evidence-informed health Policymaking (STP) 17: dealing with insufficient research evidence. *Health Research Policy and Systems* **7**, S17.

CHAPTER 12

Getting the most out of research: using what we know

Dell Horey[1], *Jessica Kaufman*[2] *and Sophie Hill*[3]
[1]Research Fellow, Division of Health Research, Faculty of Health Sciences, La Trobe University, Bundoora, Victoria, Australia
[2]Research Assistant, Cochrane Consumers and Communication Review Group, Centre for Health Communication and Participation, Australian Institute for Primary Care and Ageing, La Trobe University, Bundoora, Victoria, Australia
[3]Coordinating Editor/Head, Cochrane Consumers and Communication Review Group, Centre for Health Communication and Participation, Australian Institute for Primary Care and Ageing, La Trobe University, Bundoora, Victoria, Australia

Research evidence can encompass a seemingly boundless range of information and appears in numerous forms. It is no surprise that the people who use evidence come from similarly varied backgrounds and seek information for many different purposes.

The four primary groups of people who use health research evidence are: (1) policy makers, (2) healthcare professionals, (3) researchers and (4) consumers. Their reasons for searching may be quite different. They may be casually interested in a topic; facing a crisis or emergency that requires action; exploring care options for patients, for themselves or for a family member; undertaking a review or audit; preparing a research proposal or working on clinical practice guidelines. For all of these groups, reviews that compile evidence across individual trials and studies are valuable sources of information.

We already know a lot

The newest study does not necessarily provide the best research. As Richard Light and David Pillemer argue, 'Novelty in and of itself is shallow without links to the past. It is possible to evaluate an innovation

The Knowledgeable Patient: Communication and Participation in Health – A Cochrane Handbook, First Edition.
Edited by Sophie Hill.

only by comparisons with its predecessors' [1]. This is why the literature review – and in particular the systematic review – is such a valuable tool for those in search of research evidence. Systematic reviews synthesise the research that has already been done on a topic, and can provide new insight and a more complete picture than each isolated study. The information contained in such reviews can be utilised by a wide variety of audiences.

There is no guarantee that evidence synthesised in a systematic review will lead to a clear conclusion. However, this does not make the review any less useful. As Light and Pillemer suggest, disagreements between research findings offer a valuable opportunity for the reader. Divergent outcomes may result from carrying out the same intervention in different settings, from an intervention being implemented differently or even different interventions sharing the same name. Exploring conflicting findings may teach the reader how to implement an intervention in their setting successfully in the future [1].

This chapter looks at examples of how Cochrane reviews can provide evidence that is relevant to different audiences and how that evidence can be used by them. It proposes four theoretical scenarios facing a policy maker, health professional, researcher and consumer. Users of evidence may be confronted by different findings from systematic reviews – the intervention does not work as expected, the research is still ambivalent in its key messages or the intervention may be subject to widespread variation in practice. These scenarios are explored by showing readers of Cochrane reviews what else they can find beyond the 'bottom line' of the review.

Cochrane systematic reviews

The Cochrane Library contains more than 5500 peer-reviewed bodies of work, including over 3600 Cochrane systematic reviews of effectiveness and nearly 2000 Cochrane protocols. These reviews bring together the highest quality research evidence in a broad range of health topics and are primarily concerned with the effects of health interventions. Each Cochrane intervention review asks whether particular interventions work compared with their alternatives. While there is not always sufficient evidence, or evidence of sufficient quality, to answer a specific question about the effectiveness of interventions, Cochrane reviews are important sources of information in other ways.

Cochrane reviews synthesise existing research. This is not as straightforward as it might seem, particularly when complex interventions are involved, but it is probably one of the most important attributes of Cochrane reviews for all audiences as it shows how to make sense of the available research. This is particularly valuable when a topic has been approached in a different way or when there is no clear conceptual framework guiding research in a new area.

Cochrane authors are strongly encouraged to identify any data in the studies included in the review which signal potential or real harms associated with the intervention.

See Table 8.1 (in Chapter 8) for an explanation of what is contained in each section of a Cochrane review.

Using what we know

Health policy makers

A health policy maker must prepare a report for the Health Department, examining the effectiveness of patient contracts in changing health behaviour.

The policy maker carried out a deliberate search and found a Cochrane systematic review on the topic 'Contracts between patients and healthcare practitioners for improving patients' adherence to treatment, prevention and health promotion activities' by Xavier Bosch-Capblanch and colleagues [2].

Contracts are agreements made by consumers – either with themselves, their healthcare provider or carer – that commit the consumer to a particular behaviour or set of behaviours, usually with the aim of helping follow treatment requirements. Bosch-Capblanch and colleagues looked at studies where contracts were made between consumers and healthcare providers to improve adherence to treatment, or adopt prevention or health promotion activities. The final review included 30 randomised controlled trials (RCTs), most poorly designed or poorly reported. One-third of the included trials were concerned with behaviour relating to addictions, four with hypertension, three with weight control and the remaining 13 with a mix of health promotion, prevention and treatment goals. Results were mixed. Half of the studies favoured the use of the contracts for at least one outcome, but six trials favoured the control group. Overall, the majority of trials showed no difference between those that used contracts and those that did not.

Despite the lack of conclusive findings, the Bosch-Capblanch review still offered useful information to the policy maker. For instance, it describes possible ethical issues arising from contract implementation, noting in particular the danger that arises when a patient's access to care is dependent on their contracted behaviour. In Section 'Implications for Practice' , the authors indicate that contracts may have positive effects for certain treatment situations such as substance addiction, but in some cases contracts may also be harmful. The uncertainty of beneficial outcomes means that the policy maker will likely suggest that the Health Department support more proven interventions for their population.

The review also describes the features of contracts and explains that contingency contracts include conditional rewards, which, like penalties, are only directed at consumers in those contracts reported in the literature. Health providers do not receive any additional benefit for their role in a contract, nor are there penalties if they fail to meet their side of the contract terms. This approach indicates thinking which is not supportive of shared decision-making – instead all responsibility is placed onto consumers. Understanding this aspect of a contract approach may assist the policy maker to frame the relevance of the evidence within an existing policy context. For instance, in Australia the Victorian Department of Health is running a campaign that supports shared decision-making, through its strategic policy, 'Doing it with us not for us' [3].

The Bosch-Capblanch review is also useful in other ways. It gives information on the type of options available through contracts by describing the types of activities required and the incentives or punishments used to encourage the desired behaviour change among those studies included in the review. In addition, the review includes a summary of known barriers and enablers of adherence to treatment regimens, helping policy makers understand the broader context for the use of contracts and other strategies used to change health behaviours.

Health professionals

A health professional at a specialist cancer hospital has been asked to undertake a review and audit of the role of breast care nurses (BCNs) in improving outcomes for breast cancer patients.

The health professional searched *The Cochrane Library* and found a relevant review by Susanne Cruickshank and colleagues: 'Specialist breast care nurses for supportive care of women with breast cancer' [4].

The Cochrane review of this intervention identified five relevant RCTs involving over 1000 women, yet found limited evidence to support the role because of significant heterogeneity (i.e. diversity) across the different studies [4]. The studies varied in two main ways: (1) the roles undertaken by the nurses were different and (2) the studies used different outcome measures, suggesting conflicting understandings of the possible impact of this role. Differences in how the study populations or data were reported in terms of age or stage of breast cancer were also apparent. The review concluded that sufficient evidence from three trials showed that BCNs appeared to have some positive effects on quality of life in the short term, but this was difficult to distinguish from the impact of the multidisciplinary care team generally.

This review is an example of evidence in which results are not certain. However, reviews with uncertain results, regardless of their conclusions or lack thereof, can also be valuable for a health professional because they collect and assess all the evidence on a given subject. When confronted with the huge quantity and variable quality of available research, it may be tempting to take a short cut and use one study from a reputable journal to inform a decision. However, Mike Clarke points out that individual published studies often represent the most surprising or unusual results rather than the most common, and may overestimate or underestimate the intervention's effectiveness [5].

A health professional who looks at only a few of the individual BCN trials might have difficulty assessing their quality or comparing their results, and may reach a conclusion about the effectiveness of BCNs not actually supported by all the evidence. With a systematic review, all the available evidence is brought together in one place. Though this review shows no certain outcome for the intervention, it is preferable to know this, rather than basing future decisions and programmes on limited or poorer quality evidence.

The review also offers another valuable lesson for the health professional. It indicates that service providers should have greater input in designing and carrying out research trials in this field. The 'Implications for Research' portion of the review suggests further research should take into account the multiprofessional nature of care. The health professional consulting this review as a part of a hospital audit on BCNs could make recommendations to support or implement further research in his or her particular hospital.

Researchers

A graduate student is developing a research proposal for thesis research on peer-supported healthcare initiatives.

Researchers can use systematic reviews as a useful starting point when developing further research. Reviews summarise the topic, assess and compile current research, identify gaps in the evidence and provide a framework for approaching future research. They also describe the decisions other researchers have made, such as the definitions used, how interventions and outcomes have been categorised, the selection of comparisons and outcomes and who to include or exclude as participants.

The student begins her research by looking for a systematic review, in order to help her develop the approach she will use in conducting further research for her thesis. She finds a review by Jeremy Dale and colleagues entitled 'Peer support telephone calls for improving health' [6].

Peer support in a healthcare context is defined as 'the provision of emotional, appraisal and informational assistance by a created social network member who possesses experiential knowledge of a specific behaviour or stressor and similar characteristics as the target population' [7]. The Dale review looks at telephone peer support and describes a number of ways in which peer telephone support can vary, from who initiates the call, how peer supporters are involved, how frequently calls are made and the type of content the calls might cover. The review authors categorise content into three types: (1) emotional support, (2) appraisal support, which provides encouragement and affirmation and (3) informational support, which is 'the provision of knowledge relevant to problem-solving'.

The review included seven RCTs involving nearly 2500 participants. There were three main groups: (1) new mothers (breastfeeding and high risk of post-natal depression), (2) women aged 40 or more (mammography reminders) and (3) people with chronic health conditions (diabetes and post-heart attack). All telephone calls were initiated by the peer supporter at the outset. This implies that extending the review's findings to peer support programmes where the person receiving the peer support initiates contact may not be appropriate.

The review could not statistically combine data from the trials for meta-analysis, but a narrative presentation of the findings shows that telephone peer support achieved its intended purpose, particularly if the calls involved informational support. There was also some evidence that calls that included a combination of support (informational, appraisal and emotional) were more effective when the focus was complex behaviour change, such as encouraging breastfeeding. Emotional support alone appeared to be ineffective.

The review included information on the experience of those people providing peer support, although no studies measured any outcomes for this group. This information was collected in a qualitative stage in some of the included trials. This information extends the findings of effectiveness to understanding key issues in implementing peer support. Three studies, all involving emotional support, provided qualitative data. Three key issues were identified. First, it was important to peer supporters that they felt they had helped in some way – by giving advice, helping with problem-solving, advocating and/or lessening fears. The role was less satisfying when this did not occur. Second, sharing experiences with others was valued by peer supporters and helped form relationships between the peers. Third, sometimes peer supporters can feel vulnerable and confronted by their own anxieties.

Section 'Implications for Research' of the review provides an outline of information and suggestions to guide future researchers. For instance, Dale and colleagues recommend that future triallists 'audio record calls and conduct content analysis to discover more about the types of interchanges most effective in improving health and health-related behaviour' [6]. The review authors also indicate that more research is needed into the impact of peer support calls on peers and the receivers of support. By consulting this review before conducting her research, the graduate student is more likely to develop a study that addresses research gaps, instead of perpetuating existing insufficiencies.

Consumers

A healthcare consumer has a painful foot condition and is seeking information to help her make a treatment decision.

Healthcare consumers must make many decisions, especially with the encouragement to take a broad view of healthcare – one that spans health promotion, chronic health conditions and acute care. Some health decisions are made every day, while other decisions are less common. A simple model for health decisions incorporating three main elements provides a useful framework. Health decisions rely on personal preferences and values, the context in which a decision is made and the evidence available to inform them.

This last section looks at how consumers can use evidence available to them to inform their decisions.

The most common health decision in the research literature is concerned with treatment choice (see Chapter 8 for several stories from consumers on how they used a Cochrane review). The consumer in this example has been diagnosed with Morton's neuroma, a nerve pain that affects the toes, typically the third toe. It can be so severe that people may be cautious about walking or putting their foot to the ground. It is most common among middle-aged women. While there are no prevalence studies, it is believed to contribute significantly to orthopaedic clinic populations. The cause is not clear, but neuromas appear to be associated with the structure of a particular nerve in the foot and possible compression within the bony cavity confines around the toes. It also seems likely that wearing heeled footwear plays a part, but this is not always explicit in the health literature.

Several treatments for the condition are used: the use of insoles, corticosteroid injections and surgery on the nerve, either to remove the fibrous growths or release the pressure on the nerve. While surgery is commonly used, there are doubts about its effectiveness and concerns about complications, including possible recurrence. Steroid injection is considered a conservative alternative, at least initially, but again there is poor evidence to show that it works. Several other interventions are reported in clinical practice, but few have been adequately tested.

In their review 'Interventions for the treatment of Morton's neuroma' [8], Colin Thomson and colleagues identified four RCTs from their search of the literature. One was excluded because it did not contain sufficient information to use in the review. The other three trials involved 121 participants and used very different therapeutic approaches. One trial tested orthoses (shoe inserts), while the other two tested surgical techniques: a comparison of different management of nerve ends after re-section and comparison of removal of the nerve from either the bottom or top of the foot.

Despite the small size of the three studies (between 43 and 53 participants in each), complications were identified in each, including infections, lower limb pain and recurrence.

In Section 'Implications for Practice' of the review, the authors determined that there was insufficient evidence to assess whether surgical or non-surgical interventions for Morton's neuroma are effective. Despite the lack of a certain conclusion, the review still influenced the consumer's treatment choice. She decided to change her footwear to see if it made any difference before embarking on a treatment that may not work. She now only wears flat shoes, and while the pain has not entirely disappeared, it occurs infrequently and is manageable.

Conclusion

Cochrane reviews are rich sources of information for many different audiences. They are an efficient way of using research knowledge gained in the past to bring it into present decision-making contexts. Reviews are more than the 'bottom line' of an effectiveness statement. They contain a wealth of detailed information about the interventions used (and the comparison controls), the type of people included in the trials, the outcomes which were assessed, information about possible harms and information about the theories and concepts underlying the research. The structured nature of Cochrane reviews allows readers to go to the authors' conclusions for practice and research and to benefit from the insights the authors have gained from the review process.

References

1. Light R, Pillemer D (1984) *Summing Up*. Harvard University Press, Cambridge, MA.
2. Bosch-Capblanch X, Abba K, Prictor M, Garner P (2007) Contracts between patients and healthcare practitioners for improving patients' adherence to treatment, prevention and health promotion activities. *Cochrane Database of Systematic Reviews*, CD004808.
3. Victorian Government (2009) *Doing it with us not for us: strategic direction 2010–13*. Rural and Regional Health and Aged Care Services Division Victorian Government Department of Health, Melbourne. Available from: http://www.health.vic.gov.au/consumer/downloads/strategic_direction_2010-13.pdf. Accessed: 18 February 2010.
4. Cruickshank S, Kennedy C, Lockhart K, Dosser I, Dallas L (2008) Specialist breast care nurses for supportive care of women with breast cancer. *Cochrane Database of Systematic Reviews*, CD005634.
5. Clarke M (2004) Doing new research? Don't forget the old. *Public Library of Science Medicine* **1**, 100–102.
6. Dale J, Caramlau IO, Lindenmeyer A, Williams SM (2008) Peer support telephone calls for improving health. *Cochrane Database of Systematic Reviews*, CD006903.
7. Dennis C, Hodnett E, Gallop R, Chalmers B (2002) The effect of peer support on breast-feeding duration among primiparous women: a randomized controlled trial. *Canadian Medical Association Journal* **166**, 21–28.
8. Thomson CE, Martin D, Gibson JNA (2004) Interventions for the treatment of Morton's neuroma. *Cochrane Database of Systematic Reviews*, CD003118.

CHAPTER 13

Research agendas for knowledgeable patients

Ruth Stewart[1] *and Sandy Oliver*[2]

[1]ESRC Research Fellow, Social Science Research Unit, Institute of Education, University of London, London, United Kingdom

[2]Professor of Public Policy, Social Science Research Unit and EPPI-Centre, Institute of Education, University of London, London, United Kingdom

Introduction

This chapter starts by considering how research is funded and the opportunities this presents for involving patients and the wider public in deciding what problems deserve research and how that research should be done. It then draws on a number of UK and international examples to describe:

- Public involvement in research, why it is important and how it might increase the relevance and applicability of research.
- The background to public involvement (using the United Kingdom as a case study), different methods of involvement and the impacts of such involvement on research.
- What can be done to enhance public involvement in research and the key parameters that need to be considered.

In discussing involvement in research, this chapter uses particular terminology. Across health areas and settings, the terms used to describe the people involved vary widely, with different conventions depending on the region and discipline. Terms include patient, public, user, consumer, carer, lay person and citizen [1]. In line with the title of this book, we consider primarily the interests of patients. However, patients are part of a wider public and the concept of involvement is equally applicable to carers, service users who are not ill and the wider public – all of whom may bring or use knowledge for decisions about health services and products.

The Knowledgeable Patient: Communication and Participation in Health – A Cochrane Handbook, First Edition. Edited by Sophie Hill.

Why public involvement is important

The importance of evidence-informed decision-making and the value of systematic reviews have been established in Chapters 2, 8 and 12. Systematic reviews provide a way of drawing together current best evidence for patients to share decisions about their care with their health professionals, confident that the evidence they have is the best available, where 'best' is seen in terms of technical rigour. The growth of systematic reviews and evidence-informed health has been paralleled by the growth of public involvement in guiding research and policy. These two movements need to combine so that systematic reviews are seen as the best available evidence in terms of relevance to patients' own concerns as well as rigour.

Public involvement in health research and science is generally justified by several arguments. First, a consideration of ethics, human rights and citizenship justifies public involvement in choosing which areas of life deserve research to alleviate the most serious problems. It also ensures the accountability of researchers who are addressing these problems. Second, debates about science and society are often framed to seek public support for science and technology by focusing on material and financial benefits – the key goals in advanced knowledge-based market economies. Third, pragmatic arguments that anticipate better research, better use of research findings and, ultimately, improved health are used to justify the involvement of specific groups of patients, carers or service users in deciding how the research should be conducted.

These arguments all apply to health services research programmes where there is growing public involvement in the hope that specific research projects will be more relevant, more ethical or the research findings or scientific developments will be more beneficial or readily used.

Public and political support for health services research is valuable at a national level too. Capacity for high-quality research in the United Kingdom's National Health Service (NHS), for example, attracts research and development funding from the pharmaceutical, devices and biotechnology industries. These industries are prime investors and form a major part of the United Kingdom's knowledge economy. The pharmaceutical industry alone accounts for 25% of the United Kingdom's business investment in R&D and it is a significant employer of highly skilled staff [2].

Public involvement for a national research agenda

Funding for research comes from a range of sources: mostly industry, but also governments, and some from charities [2]. In the United Kingdom, public funding has been accompanied by a long history of public involvement in research agenda setting. This was heralded by the launch of the NHS Research and Development strategy in 1991 and the introduction of a 'systematic approach to identifying and setting R&D priorities in which NHS staff and the users of the Service [were] asked to identify important issues which confront[ed] them and, in partnership with the research community, to characterise and prioritise these problems as the basis for seeking solutions' [3]. This was followed in 1996 by the Department of Health, establishing the Standing Advisory Group for Consumer Involvement in Research and Development (now called INVOLVE – www.invo.org.uk) to develop and support public involvement in R&D. In 2003, after publication of 'Clinical Trials for Tomorrow' [4], the Medical Research Council and the Department of Health funded the James Lind Initiative to promote public and professional knowledge about, and engagement with, clinical trials (www.lindalliance.org). As one of the initiatives taken under the aegis of the James Lind Initiative, the James Lind Alliance was launched in 2004 to foster collaboration between patients and clinicians in 'working partnerships' to identify research priorities addressing uncertainties about the effects of treatments. The alliance now leads the way in the United Kingdom in engaging patients and clinicians together to identify and prioritise the questions that they agree are most important and that have not yet been addressed by a rigorous systematic review.

Public involvement for international research agendas

Systematic reviews have a pivotal role in determining the direction of research: they highlight where the evidence is sufficiently strong and where there are gaps. The international Cochrane Collaboration is central to the production of systematic reviews worldwide. The Collaboration has a number of avenues through which consumers can contribute to research priorities. Consumers and consumer organisations are invited to tell Cochrane Review Groups about interventions and questions that are important to them and that they would like to see reviewed or invited to identify specific topics [5]. At various stages of the review development process, consumers can give feedback on the relevance of the review question, comment on the review itself or identify outcomes that are important to them [1]. Lastly, within the Collaboration is an entity – the Cochrane Consumer Network – which exists 'to enable and support consumers in contributing to the function of collaborative review groups and other Cochrane entities'. The Network offers 'communication with other consumers and groups, a sense of belonging, links with consumer and patient groups, and dissemination of information from Cochrane reviews' [6].

Numerous countries now have public policies which support forms of public involvement in research agenda setting. A recent systematic review of research identified examples of clinicians and patients working together to set research agendas in the USA, Australia, the United Kingdom, the Netherlands and Zambia [7]. These activities cut across mental health, breast cancer, dementia, chronic obstructive pulmonary disease (COPD), maternity care, HIV/AIDS, child welfare, and faecal and urinary incontinence. This spread of activity suggests that it is some of the greatest burdens and most intractable problems that have galvanised patients and clinicians to work together.

An example of this is the global spread of HIV/AIDS which prompted an innovative exercise in Zambia in which patients and carers, clinicians and other health professionals worked together to identify research questions in HIV/AIDS [8]. Participants included representatives from the Zambia Network of People Living with HIV/AIDS and international HIV clinicians, as well as researchers from medical institutions, members of the Ministry of Health, National AIDS Council staff, representatives of non-government organisations and members of the public media. Following presentations on the pressing issues in HIV/AIDS in Zambia, six intensive small-group discussions resulted in six major research priorities. These included questions relating to clinical decisions, such as when to initiate highly active antiretroviral therapy (HAART) in relation to $CD4^+$ cell count (a measure used to determine when to begin treatment for HIV-infected patients), and others considering more social issues, such as the need to assess strategies for maximising adherence to antiretroviral therapy in Zambia.

Research funding models and public involvement

Whilst research priorities vary worldwide, the models for public involvement in agenda setting fit within a broad framework, dependent in part on the approach to research funding. Sometimes public and charitable funders decide what research they want done and then advertise for teams to undertake the research. This is called commissioned research, and it usually addresses precise questions that organisations want answered. Alternatively, funds are made available through responsive research programmes on more general topics, and teams are invited to respond by proposing promising topics or questions they would like to address. In both the cases, decisions are informed by expert review, where the relevance and rigour of proposals are assessed independently.

Within these funding arrangements, the first opportunity for patient or public influence is at the stage of setting the scope of the research: broad topics encompassing important health burdens for responsive programmes, and narrow topics or even precise questions for commissioned programmes. The second opportunity for patient influence in both these types of programmes is at the stage of research proposals: research teams may elicit patients' views when developing their proposals, and the funders may elicit patients' views when assessing the proposals.

In practice, funders may vary from involving patients at all stages of the decision-making process to little or no involvement [9].

A broad framework for public involvement

As a part of traditional social research, researchers may invite patients to share their *views and experiences on health, health services or health services research.* These views can be communicated in person or in written reports or academic papers. In many cases, patients have more to say about health and health services – which they may interact with frequently – than health services research – which they may encounter only occasionally. This means that researchers first need to interpret patient statements about health or health services in order to relate them to topics that can be addressed in research. Then, researchers and research commissioners can analyse the collected patient statements in order to *prioritise* future research.

Alternatively, patients can be consulted directly about their *priorities for research.* In these cases, patients are made aware that their views will be used to shape a decision, even though they are not involved in making the decision. In the case of responsive research programmes, research teams applying for funds can take it upon themselves to elicit patients' priorities for research and reflect these in their applications; some funders encourage such efforts. Within commissioned research programmes, the funders can elicit patients' priorities and then commission research to address these priorities: a recent survey found this last approach was uncommon [9].

The most common means by which patients are consulted about their priorities for research is through the process of expert review of research proposals or funding applications. For both commissioned and responsive programmes, patients can be engaged in the review process and offer opinions on the value of the research from their perspective. When asked to review funding applications, public and scientific reviewers tend to be asked to review different aspects of the research applications and are sometimes involved in different stages of the funding selection process – the stage at which the public comment on applications can shape their scope to influence decisions; for example, the United Kingdom's Alzheimer's Society first invites their network of specially recruited carers to comment on applications, and only those which carers consider most important are sent out to scientists for a second phase of expert review.

Patients and the public can also be invited to *share in the decision-making process.* This level of involvement requires more collaborative partnerships.

Collaborative partnerships for shared decision-making

Patients and the public can be involved in decision-making about research priorities in a number of different ways, sometimes using a two-step process whereby people have been engaged first in homogeneous groups, before debating issues or priorities within a mixed group of stakeholders. This approach to collaboration has the advantage of allowing people to share their views in a more familiar, potentially less challenging environment first, before any cross-disciplinary discussion takes place. In a recent Dutch study, this approach was used to involve patients and carers, clinicians and other health professionals, as well as researchers and scientists, to identify research questions in COPD, asthma and kidney disease [10]. Professionals were drawn from a variety of disciplines including biomedical, social, clinical and epidemiological science. Different stakeholder groups first identified their own research priorities and then the mixed group of 24 stakeholders met to identify a shared list of highest priority questions. Whilst there are arguments for the approach described above, and forcing mixed groups to discuss issues from the beginning is thought to identify a wider range of potential issues, reaching a consensus is much more difficult [11].

Another important aspect of engaging patients and clinicians collaboratively in prioritising research agendas is the means by which the decisions are made. This can vary from informal to more formalised methods such as voting, scoring, and using consensus conferences or multistage initiatives such as Delphi studies.Voting is a simple one-step way of gathering participants' views to inform a decision without the need for successive rounds. Scoring goes one step further. Participants are asked to indicate the relative preference for topics or questions for research. In the NHS, a scoring approach was used to identify issues and prioritise research questions in relation to the interface between primary and secondary care [12]. Initially, an advisory group including nurses, doctors, managers, researchers and patients met to determine topics for R&D funding. The advisory group then formed three panels to consider three main topics. Each panel reviewed existing evidence, considered responses to large-scale consultations and identified key issues to forward to the advisory group. Twenty-one topics were agreed and scored by all members of the group from highest to lowest priority to produce a list of topics in priority order.

More complex than voting or scoring is the Delphi technique, which involves using two or more rounds of questionnaires to gather the views of the same or a different group of individuals, using increasing levels of complexity. For instance, an initial questionnaire might gather suggestions, a second asks participants to vote on a list of topics and give reasons, and a final questionnaire might include a shortlist of ten topics drawn up by researchers following the previous round, asking participants to prioritise their top three. Each round of questionnaire enables the group to approach greater consensus. An example of this can be found in the area of primary mental healthcare [13]. A three-round Delphi exercise was used with 30 participants, including primary care nurses, general practitioners, psychiatrists, a clinical psychologist, directors of a mental health charity and users of primary care services.

Consensus conferences provide another means of reaching decisions about research priorities with patients. These involve more complex accumulation of views through discussion, but without the benefit of numerical votes or scores, they require expert facilitation to enable a decision to be reached. This method has been used effectively in identifying research priorities for faecal and urinary incontinence [14]. Initially a number of experts from all disciplines that treat incontinence were asked to identify the three most important research priorities from the perspective of their disciplines. A consensus conference was then held in which patient advocates and health professionals explored and debated the relative importance of the research priorities suggested.

All these examples are drawn from a growing literature of studies that approached patients and clinicians, either independently or together, to prioritise problems deserving research. Whilst policy and supportive initiatives can increase patient involvement in setting research agendas, the question remains: does it make a difference? Indeed, there is some concern that involving non-researchers in the process may compromise research rigour in some way [15]. There is a small and growing pool of empirical evidence for the impact of involving patients [16, 17].

Areas of patient/public influence are wide ranging and include introducing new ideas and perspectives to discussions [10]; influencing decisions about what research is funded through peer-review processes [18] and membership on funding committees [19]; changing research practice by influencing the research team [20]; and changing attitudes towards patients and towards shared decision-making [19].

Putting research into policy or practice will require...

Having reviewed the key issues within patient and public involvement in research, there are a number of lessons about how such involvement might be developed to increase the relevance and applicability of research more broadly.

Formal initiatives such as the United Kingdom's James Lind Alliance are required to enable the integration of patient involvement into research agenda setting. Furthermore, by increasing the requirement for research applications to specify patient and public involvement in the proposed studies, the scope for public influence on research is greatly increased.

Whilst public involvement in research is still relatively new, there are a growing number of initiatives throughout the world. Sharing experiences of public involvement through international networks such as the Cochrane Collaboration and collating examples of patient involvement through published bibliographies and systematic reviews of research [7,18,21] enable accumulation of knowledge about how to facilitate public involvement in research, its potential impact and limitations, and how best to evaluate these.

The impact of public involvement is limited by the scope of the involvement itself. There are a number of key factors which may shape the public's influence and these need consideration by those designing, facilitating and evaluating public involvement. These include:

- whether members of the public are asked to contribute their views as citizens (and taxpayers where research is publicly funded) or their views based on their experiences of services;
- whether participants only contribute their views or also share in decision-making;
- the extent to which individuals are informed about the research they are contributing to or the specific questions they are addressing, or both;
- the means by which they contribute;
- whether they contribute alone or in groups, and whether groups are homogeneous groups or mixed groups with researchers or clinicians;
- whether their contributions are made in private or in a public forum;
- the attention given to their contributions;
- the number of others involved and the degree of influence they have on decision-making, and their attitudes to public involvement; and
- the timing of public involvement in the decision-making process.

In addition, the theory and philosophy of public involvement needs development, as it is still unclear how much power *should* be assigned to the public in decision-making about research, and whether or not public influence should be greater than researcher or clinician influence. One argument suggests that there are particular roles for patients and clinicians (such as in setting agendas) and other roles for scientists (such as maximising research rigour).

Addressing these important issues will increase the potential for patient and public involvement in research. Through greater public involvement in research and increased understanding of this involvement, the potential exists to ensure not only that systematic reviews, as one key example of research for building knowledge, are viewed as the means to draw together current best evidence for decision-making, but that systematic reviews are also seen as the best available evidence in terms of relevance to patients' own concerns too.

References

1. Hill S (2007) Involving the consumers in health research. In: Saks M, Allsop J, (eds.) *Researching Health: Qualitative, Quantitative and Mixed Methods*. Sage Publications, London, pp. 351–367.

2. Cooksey D (2006) *A Review of UK Health Research Funding*. HM Treasury, London.
3. Department of Health, UK (1993) *Research for Health*. HMSO, London.
4. Medical Research Council (2003) *Clinical Trials for Tomorrow: An MRC Review of Randomised Control Trials*. MRC, London.
5. Buckley B, Grant A, Tincello D, Wagg A, Firkins L, (On behalf of the James Lind Alliance Priority Setting Partnership on Urinary Incontinence) (2009) Prioritising research: patients, carers and clinicians working together to identify and prioritise important clinical uncertainties in urinary incontinence. *Neurourology and Urodynamics* **29**, 708–714.
6. Cochrane Consumer Network. Available from: www.cochrane.org/consumers/homepage.htm. Accessed: 23 March 2011.
7. Stewart R, Oliver S (2008) *A Systematic Map of Studies of Patients' and Clinicians' Research Priorities*. James Lind Alliance, London.
8. Zulu I, Schuman P, Musonda R, et al. (2004) Priorities for antiretroviral therapy research in sub-Saharan Africa: a 2002 consensus conference in Zambia. *Journal of Acquired Immune Deficiency Syndromes* **36**, 831–834.
9. Staley K, Haley B (2008) *Scoping Research Priority Setting, and the Presence of Patient and Public Involvement, with UK Clinical Research Organisations and Funders*. James Lind Alliance, London.
10. Caron-Flinterman J, Broerse J, Teerling J, et al. (2006) Stakeholder participation in health research agenda setting. The case of asthma and COPD research in the Netherlands. *Science and Public Policy* **33**, 291–304.
11. Murphy MK, Black NA, Lamping DL, et al. (1998) Consensus development methods, and their use in clinical guideline development. *Health Technology Assessment* **2**, i–iv, 1–88.
12. Jones R, Lamont T, Haines A (1995) Setting priorities for research and development in the NHS: a case study on the interface between primary and secondary care. *British Medical Journal* **311**, 1076–1080.
13. James P, Aitken P, Burns T (2002) Research priorities for primary care mental health: a Delphi exercise. *Primary Care Psychiatry* **8**, 27–30.
14. Whitehead W, Wald A, Norton N (2004) Priorities for treatment research from different professional perspectives. *Gastroenterology* **126**, S180–S185.
15. Thompson J, Barber R, Ward PR, et al. (2009) Health researchers' attitudes towards public involvement in health research. *Health Expectations* **12**, 209–220.
16. Staley K (2009) *Exploring Impact: Public Involvement in NHS, Public Health and Social Care Research*. INVOLVE, Eastleigh.
17. Boote JD (2009) *Patient and Public Involvement in Health and Social Care Research: A Bibliography*. NIHR Research Design Service for Yorkshire and the Humber. Available from: http://www.rds-yh.nihr.ac.uk/patient-and-public-involvement.aspx. Accessed: 1 April 2010.
18. Oliver S (2004) Involving consumers in research and development agenda setting for the NHS: developing an evidence-based approach. *Health Technology Assessment* **8**, 154.
19. Andejeski Y, Bisceglio IT, Dickersin K, et al. (2002) Quantitative impact of including consumers in the scientific review of breast cancer research proposals. *Journal of Women's Health & Gender-based Medicine* **11**, 379–388.

20. Langston AL, McCallum M, Campbell MK, Robertson C, Ralston SH (2005) An integrated approach to consumer representation and involvement in a multicentre randomized controlled trial. *Clinical Trials* **2**, 80–87.
21. Nilsen ES, Myrhaug HT, Johansen M, Oliver S, Oxman AD (2006) Methods of consumer involvement in developing healthcare policy and research, clinical practice guidelines and patient information material. *Cochrane Database of Systematic Reviews*, CD004563.

CHAPTER 14

Managing multiple health problems: is there evidence to support consumer-focused communication and participation?

Rebecca E. Ryan[1] *and Sophie Hill*[2]
[1]Research Fellow, Cochrane Consumers and Communication Review Group, Centre for Health Communication and Participation, Australian Institute for Primary Care and Ageing, La Trobe University, Bundoora, Victoria, Australia
[2]Coordinating Editor/Head, Cochrane Consumers and Communication Review Group, Centre for Health Communication and Participation, Australian Institute for Primary Care and Ageing, La Trobe University, Bundoora, Victoria, Australia

Living with more than one health problem has attracted renewed attention, not surprisingly given that rates are rising. The proportion of people with more than one health problem (multimorbidity) is increasing and it is not just a problem associated with ageing. People with multimorbidity have complex, but poorly understood and documented, communication needs. Placing these needs at the centre of our analysis, this chapter examines what evidence exists to support the use of evidence-based interventions for communication and participation in the area of medicines where people have multimorbidity. The analysis finds little evidence, pointing to research, policy and practice challenges for the future.

What is multimorbidity?

Multimorbidity is the term used to describe having two or more conditions at the same time [1, 2]. Most commonly this refers to having more than one chronic health condition, for instance, having depression and heart disease.

The Knowledgeable Patient: Communication and Participation in Health – A Cochrane Handbook, First Edition.
Edited by Sophie Hill.

However, if we focus on how consumers manage their health, chronic illness is important, but not the only issue. Acute conditions come and go, and may compound or make coping with chronic diseases difficult. Treatments for chronic problems may create new health problems. Health promotion may also be a goal, as it is for others in the community, and opportunities to engage in healthier lifestyle will be affected by underlying health problems.

Therefore, in this chapter, the term multimorbidity is used to encompass health status that is complex and dynamic. This could mean the interaction or accumulation of more than one chronic condition, the addition of acute or short-term illness, such as flu, and altered health status over time, including both improvement and decline. Population goals associated with health promotion and screening must also be factored in.

Why is multimorbidity an issue for health systems?

Most people have more than one condition when seeking care for chronic diseases [3–5], and with rising chronic disease rates and accruing new diseases, rates of multimorbidity are likely to continue to rise. For example, nearly 80% of all Australians reported at least one long-term condition in 2004–2005 [6], with over 35% of Australians having two or more conditions [7].

Multimorbidity is often described as an issue of the ageing population as it is more common with increasing age [1]. Rates of multimorbidity do vary across disease combinations and with age [7], but more recently there has been recognition that rates are also rising among children and younger adults [5, 8, 9]. For example, some estimates suggest that up to 10% of younger people (including infants, children and adolescents up to 19 years of age) have two or more diseases [1]. This means that multimorbidity is an issue affecting people of all ages, despite being age associated.

What kinds of challenges will this raise? People with a single chronic illness face substantial challenges in managing and self-managing health [6, 10]. These grow in number and complexity when a person accrues more than one health problem. People with multiple concurrent illnesses face significantly poorer health and other outcomes than the rest of the population, including premature death, higher rates of hospitalisation, adverse events and polypharmacy, as well as poorer quality of life, psychological outcomes and physical function [4, 11–15].

Why is multimorbidity an issue for consumers and carers?

The poorer outcomes listed above translate to higher costs not only for health systems but also for individuals and families. In particular, poorer quality of life is a major consequence of multimorbidity. Recent data from

Table 14.1 National policy frameworks: arthritis, multimorbidity and communication issues in the social domain.

USA [17]	Arthritis and other chronic diseases raise issues of social equity: there are issues that specifically affect the uninsured or underinsured, those who are disabled, have low educational levels, the unskilled workforce and other vulnerable groups
	Arthritis has a significant effect on quality of life for individuals and families
Canada [18]	People with arthritis must be enabled to participate in the life roles of importance to them (such as employment and education, social roles, personal relationships, leisure activities)
	Participation has been under-represented as an outcome in arthritis, and the impact of interventions aiming to improve participation have typically been neglected
Australia [19]	Lower socio-economic status and higher levels of risk behaviours may predispose Aboriginal and Torres Strait Islander peoples to the development of multiple conditions
	People in rural and remote areas face barriers to healthcare and support

a large American study of quality of life amongst 21,133 people with a wide range of chronic illnesses reported that people with more than one health problem had poorer quality of life and that this continued to decline as illnesses accumulated [16]. The authors reported that 'the magnitude of difference between those with multiple conditions compared with a single condition was greater ... than the difference between those with a single condition and no conditions' (p. 1201).

In Table 14.1, we present an assessment from the American, Canadian and Australian National Service Frameworks of the social burden of arthritis [17–19]. Arthritis is recognised as a major chronic disease associated with a significant burden for individuals, families and communities internationally. Arthritis co-occurs with many acute and chronic diseases, affects people from birth to old age and entails a heavy burden of self-management and disability [13, 20, 21]. National policy frameworks and action plans identify the range of issues arising for people with arthritis, for their doctors and health systems, prioritise their impact and formulate ways of meeting identified needs to improve the quality of care and health outcomes. The frameworks highlight the impact of poorer health status, lower incomes or poorer access to care on those with chronic diseases. There is recognition that having arthritis impacts adversely on people in terms of roles and opportunities in life and quality of life and that these impacts are unfairly distributed.

Acknowledging the range of problems faced by people with multimorbidity, several researchers have suggested that the way to improve outcomes in these people is to move towards patient-centred models of care for multimorbidity. This would enable tailored, individualised care to be delivered to people with complex health problems and would help to overcome the problems faced by fragmentary care organised around services rather than patients [15, 22–25]. However to move towards these models of care, it is necessary to understand better exactly what challenges and burdens are experienced by patients with multimorbidity, their carers and health professionals.

Why and how is multimorbidity an issue for communication and participation?

The burdens of multimorbidity increase both the number and the complexity of interactions people will have in managing their health [8]. But what are these burdens and how do they link to the interactions people experience and manage? Until recently, these burdens have been poorly described, or have remained largely hidden, even though the poor outcomes of multimorbidity have been well documented. More recently, it has been possible to tease out the range of different issues for people with multimorbidity. One approach to doing this has been by using an investigative framework for examining the communication issues that happen at the interconnections between research, clinical care and social life for people with multimorbidity [26, 27].

In the following section, the major communication areas are described, and the types of issues or burdens for people with multimorbidity are identified by using the investigative framework as a tool to unpack each area.

Accumulating diagnoses

If someone has more than one illness, it is only logical that they will have more to manage and that conditions and associated treatments may conflict, interact and add burdens to living, such as cost, health appointments, side effects and possibly more visits to hospital [23].

The experience of multimorbidity is also mediated by socio-economic context (e.g. income, employment and health literacy) in addition to family circumstances of caring for children or parents [3]. Poorer health status and higher use of health services are linked to poorer communication outcomes, which in turn leads to poorer health outcomes.

Deficits in the patient centredness of care, poor communication with consumers and low health literacy are pervasive problems associated with adverse events and poor health outcomes that are recognised and documented internationally [28–30]. Research suggests that people with multimorbidity may be further disadvantaged when it comes to communication in health. Prescribing physicians, for example, communicate better about newly prescribed medicines to patients with fewer co-occurring conditions [31]. People with the most complex health issues – those most likely to be following complex treatment regimens – may therefore be the ones missing out on the information and support they need. Other research indicates that patients with more co-occurring conditions rate their doctor's communication less highly than patients who are healthier [32], and that communication with doctors is a concern for many people with multimorbidity [25].

Further, expected or unexpected variations in a chronic disease over a person's lifetime, or acute exacerbations due to short-term problems such as the common cold, may present major challenges for management by health professionals, consumers and carers. Preventive care, proactive management or optimisation of treatment may take a back seat in the face of a complex set of health problems that change over time and take time and energy in clinical encounters between patients and their doctors.

Prioritisation of treatment and management decisions

Information to enable people to self-manage the symptoms of a chronic disease is critical, but where more than one disease coexists, there may be more symptoms to be managed at any given point in time; symptoms may be more severe; management of one symptom may need to be prioritised above another; or there may be conflicting advice on managing symptoms arising from different diseases or different healthcare professionals [25].

Consumers and doctors may have different treatment priorities and discussing these may be difficult. For example, a patient's priority might be managing medicines in order to minimise symptoms or side effects of medicines in order to keep working or keep up with family commitments. In comparison, a doctor's first priority might be managing an acute health problem or risk factors for future disease. Recognising that these priorities could be different and communicating about them may not always be easy where multiple diseases coexist.

Priorities may also change over a person's lifetime and these may need to be explained and negotiated with doctors. For someone with arthritis, for example, health goals when studying at a university, when trying to get pregnant, when running a business or when retired may be different. People may also have difficulty recognising or prioritising their own health concerns and so need assistance with this [15, 33]. Multiple co-occurring diseases may therefore introduce multiple competing demands [32], and determining how to prioritise and negotiate these will affect both consumers and health professionals.

Decision-making

Accumulating health problems mean that both the patient and the doctor must deal with a growing list of problems, treatments and potential interactions, and that this complexity will often from necessity form a key focus of the clinical encounter [32]. The potential for adverse events may increase, and choices may become more difficult. For example, the co-occurrence of diseases may lead to greater uncertainties associated with different choices or options [34]. There may be less evidence that is applicable when multimorbidity exists, or the goals and trade-offs of treatment may change with accumulating diseases, reflecting clinical complexity. Any or all of these possibilities may come into play with accumulating diseases, and in such situations, it may be difficult for patients to make informed choices about their health or for health professionals to convey enough information about choices and uncertainty for patients to make an informed choice [27, 32]. It is not yet clear which ways of reaching decisions are best suited to people with multimorbidity, but involving patients in shared decision-making is still critical.

Coordination

Healthcare professionals caring for people with chronic health problems may face several challenges [8, 22]. For example, the need to tailor self-management plans to individuals and their circumstances may be desirable [34], but how is this to be achieved? For people with multimorbidity, whose care may involve several different healthcare providers, the way to align different treatment strategies targeting different diseases may not be at all straightforward [15, 24]. There may not be information readily available to assist or support doctors and others to make such decisions, particularly when care plans are complex, changing over time or happening in more than one care setting. Established processes for communication between professionals may not adequately support collaborative care models, enable optimisation of treatment strategies across diseases, promote preventive care, allow the provision of information and support to patients, or even allow directly contraindicated treatments or self-management plans to be detected and associated adverse events avoided. These issues and others represent significant challenges for health professionals and health systems.

Self-management

Effective self-management of chronic conditions includes a complex range of processes or activities that must be adaptive in order to respond to changes over time [25, 33]. This includes information, skills and motivation on the part of the consumer, and the availability of education and support to assist people in self-management. The task of self-management is complex even for a single disease. With accumulating diseases, the complexity of self-management for consumers – alone and in partnership with health professionals – is likely to rise [27].

Various social and contextual factors should also be considered in relation to self-management. For instance, people with poorer health literacy may find it challenging to deal with accumulating diagnoses or manage multiple treatments regimes, and may require higher levels of support, time or simplified information. The cost and availability of care are an issue. Families may need to be more actively kept in a communication loop, rather than brought in only when there is a crisis or major decision to be made. Existing inequalities in health also need careful consideration, as an emphasis on self-care and self-management may lead to further disadvantage [35].

Information sources

At present, research evidence and the information materials derived from it for both doctors and consumers principally focus on one disease and largely ignore the interaction of diseases in patients' lives [33]. This means that there may be little or no information for patients with multimorbidity to support treatment, self-management or other health actions [25, 27, 36]. There may also be little information that is suitable for doctors to share with their patients when multimorbidity is present. A further problem arises because it is not possible to simply apply what is known from research and information derived from single diseases to people with multimorbidity [12, 24].

What does the evidence say? Multimorbidity and evidence-based management of medicines

Multimorbidity has been shown to create a heavy burden of illness and treatment for consumers and carers, reflected in a range of poorer outcomes than for others in the community. One area where people with multimorbidity may experience particular trouble is around polypharmacy (using multiple medicines) and high rates of associated adverse events [25, 27, 33, 36]. The high burden of treatment and decision-making for consumers and carers in relation to multimorbidity creates an environment in which it is difficult to manage medicines and where medicine-related adverse events and poor care coordination can flourish.

Ideally, interventions to promote safer, more effective use of medicines by consumers could help to diminish many of these problems. This might include interventions to promote better understanding of medicines and medicine taking, support people to take medicines safely and effectively, improve medicines self-management skills or minimise harms associated with using medicines (see intervention taxonomy in Chapter 3).

To investigate whether and how well the research base supporting this range of interventions on consumers' medicines use applies to people with multimorbidity, we conducted an analysis of a large database of systematic reviews of interventions to improve the prescribing and use of medicines [37]. We selected systematic reviews of interventions directed to consumers and assessed the extent to which these reviews and their included studies considered multimorbidity. The data set (n = 53) was derived from reviews published on the Cochrane Database of

Systematic Reviews and Database of Abstracts of Reviews of Effects up to September 2008, which is collected and presented within the Canadian *Rx for Change* database (www.cadth.ca/index.php/en/compus/optimal-ther-resources/interventions, under 'Consumer').

Of the 53 systematic reviews we assessed, the vast majority (45/53, 85%) did not explicitly consider multimorbidity, either at the review level or at the level of the included study. In the remaining eight reviews, people with multimorbidity were not explicitly excluded, but were typically considered in only a minority of the studies. Furthermore, while inclusion might imply interest in or some focus on multimorbidity, in fact, there was little discussion of the impact of multimorbidity on medicines use in this small subset of reviews.

The one exception to this was the issue of polypharmacy in the elderly, which was addressed in some detail by a small number of reviews. However, there is almost no evidence to guide action on the issue of complex medicines regimens beyond this age group, despite rising chronic disease and multimorbidity rates across all age groups. This means that although many interventions exist which might theoretically be able to help improve medicines use in multimorbidity, the reality is that the research evidence that evaluates these strategies does not consider, in most cases, issues of the growing number and complexity of medicines for multimorbidity. This means we have almost no research evidence to guide practice or policy on medicines in multimorbidity even though multimorbidity is a known risk factor for medicine-related adverse events [38].

What are the implications for health professionals, health policy, consumers and carers?

The analysis indicates a growing misalignment between strategies to promote informed consumers and carers, capable of self-care and informed decision-making, and the evidence base on which such strategies rest. The reviews represent a subset of evidence in one area where it could be expected that multimorbidity would be a focus – given the likelihood that many people are on multiple medicines and that a large research base exists on consumers' medicines use [39].

This gap is perhaps not surprising, given that research more widely into the effectiveness of clinical treatments and health service approaches does not consider the issues for people with multimorbidity. Various researchers have documented that research has explicitly excluded people with coexisting conditions or ignored or failed to report details of interacting health problems [3, 12, 15]. This means that the research evidence – and resources built from it, such as clinical practice guidelines and health information websites – typically only apply directly to people with a single disease. This is problematic for people with multimorbidity because of the issues raised above.

The implications are that clinicians, consumers or their family carers are left with little guidance on how to apply and discuss research findings, treatment options, medicines interactions, uncertainty or how to best manage health and balance competing priorities where multimorbidity is present. This creates a significant burden of decision-making for consumers and carers, their doctors and other health professionals, and health information providers. The other implication of research focusing on single, rather than multiple, disease(s) is that research largely ignores the interactions of diseases in people's lives where multimorbidity is present. Therefore, relatively little is known about the competing demands of managing more than one disease and how these contribute to the poor outcomes associated with multimorbidity.

The communication problems arising in relation to multimorbidity may be many and affect health consumers, professionals and systems across the interface of the clinical and social domains [26]. The rising rates of multimorbidity across all ages and the high impact of multimorbidity on health and other outcomes mean that multimorbidity will continue to be a growing concern for all parties. Research into health systems improvements for people with multimorbidity will become a priority in the next decade and research into the interconnection of clinical care and social life should be a key part of this work.

References

1. Van Den Akker M, Buntinx F, Knottnerus A (1996) Comorbidity or multimorbidity: what's in a name? A review of the literature. *European Journal of General Practice* **2**, 65–70.
2. Valderas JM, Starfield B, Sibbald B, Salisbury C, Roland M (2009) Defining comorbidity: implications for understanding health and health services. *Annals of Family Medicine* **7**, 357–363.
3. Starfield B (2003) Threads and yarns: weaving the tapestry of comorbidity. *Annals of Family Medicine* **4**, 101–103.
4. Fortin M, Hudon C, Bayliss EA, Soubhi H, Lapointe L (2007) Caring for body and soul: the importance of recognizing and managing psychological distress in persons with multimorbidity. *International Journal of Psychiatry in Medicine* **37**, 1–9.
5. Fortin M, Bravo G, Hudon C, Vanasse A, Lapointe L (2005) Prevalence of multimorbidity among adults seen in family practice. *Annals of Family Medicine* **3**, 223–228.
6. Australian Institute of Health and Welfare (2009) *Chronic Disease and Participation in Work*. Australian Institute of Health and Welfare, Canberra. Available from: http://search.aihw.gov.au/search?q=chronic%20disease%20incidence&sort=date%3AD%3AL%3Ad1&oe=UTF-8&ie=UTF-8&output=xml_no_dtd&client=default_frontend&proxystylesheet=default_frontend&site=publication_collection. Accessed: 13 July 2009.
7. Britt HC, Harrison CM, Miller GC, Knox SA (2008) Prevalence and patterns of multimorbidity in Australia. *Medical Journal of Australia* **189**, 72–77.

8. Smith SM, Ferede A, O'Dowd T (2008) Multimorbidity in younger deprived patients: an exploratory study of research and service implications in general practice. *BMC Family Practice* **9**, 6.
9. Fortin MHC, Haggerty J, Akker M, Almirall J (2010) Prevalence estimates of multimorbidity: a comparative study of two sources. *BMC Health Services Research* **10**, 111.
10. Townsend A, Wyke S, Hunt K (2006) Self-managing and managing self: practical and moral dilemmas in accounts of living with chronic illness. *Chronic Illness* **2**, 185–194.
11. Fortin M, Bravo G, Hudon C, et al. (2006) Relationship between multimorbidity and health-related quality of life of patients in primary care. *Quality of Life Research* **15**, 83–91.
12. Boyd CM, Darer J, Boult C, Fried LP, Boult L, Wu AW (2005) Clinical practice guidelines and quality of care for older patients with multiple comorbid diseases: implications for pay for performance. *Journal of the American Medical Association* **294**, 716–724.
13. Australian Institute of Health and Welfare (2010) *Arthritis and Musculoskeletal Conditions*. Australian Institute of Health and Welfare, Canberra. Available from: http://www.aihw.gov.au/nhpa/arthritis/index.cfm. Accessed: 7 October 2010.
14. Smith SM, Soubhi H, Fortin M, Hudon C, O'Dowd T (2007) Interventions to improve outcomes in patients with multimorbidity in primary care and community settings (Protocol). *Cochrane Database of Systematic Reviews*, CD006560.
15. Bayliss EA, Edwards AE, Steiner JF, Main DS (2008) Processes of care desired by elderly patients with multimorbidities. *Family Practice* **25**, 287–293.
16. Rothrock NE, Hays RD, Spritzer K, Yount SE, Riley W, Cella D (2010) Relative to the general US population, chronic diseases are associated with poorer health-related quality of life as measured by the Patient-Reported Outcomes Measurement Information System (PROMIS). *Journal of Clinical Epidemiology* **63**, 1195–1204.
17. Arthritis Foundation, Association of State and Territorial Officials, Centres for Disease Control and Prevention (1999) *The National Arthritis Action Plan: A Public Health Strategy*. Centres for Disease Control and Prevention, USS. Available from: http://www.cdc.gov/arthritis/about_us.htm. Accessed: 17 December 2008.
18. Alliance for the Canadian Arthritis Program (2006) *Report from the Summit on Standards for Arthritis Prevention and Care. November 1–2, 2005*. Ottawa, Canada. Available from: http://www.arthritisalliance.ca/home/index.html. Accessed: 22 June 2009.
19. National Health Priority Action Council (NHPAC) (2006) *National Service Improvement Framework for Osteoarthritis, Rheumatoid Arthritis and Osteoporosis*. Australian Government Department of Health and Ageing, Canberra. Available from: www.health.gov.au/internet/main/publishing.nsf/Content/pq-ncds-arthritis. Accessed: 17 December 2008.
20. Australian Institute of Health and Welfare (2010) *When Musculoskeletal Conditions and Mental Disorders Occur Together*. Australian Institute of Health and Welfare, Canberra. Available from: http://www.aihw.gov.au/publications/index.cfm/title/11155. Accessed: 10 October 2010.
21. National Arthritis and Musculoskeletal Conditions Advisory Group (NAMSCAG) (2004) *Evidence to Support the National Action Plan for Osteoarthritis, Rheumatoid Arthritis and Osteoporosis: Opportunities to Improve Health-Related Quality of Life and*

Reduce the Burden of Disease and Disability. Australian Government Department of Health and Ageing, Canberra. Available from: http://www.nhpac.gov.au/. Accessed: 7 October 2010.

22. Fortin M, Soubhi H, Hudon C, Bayliss EA, Van Den Akker M (2007) Multimorbidity's many challenges. *British Medical Journal* **334**, 1016–1017.
23. May C, Montori VM, Mair FS (2009) We need minimally disruptive medicine. *British Medical Journal* **339**, b2803.
24. van Weel C (2006) Comorbidity and guidelines: conflicting interests. Comment. *Lancet* **367**, 550–551.
25. Noel PH, Frueh BC, Larme AC, Pugh JA (2005) Collaborative care needs and preferences of primary care patients with multimorbidity. *Health Expectations* **8**, 54–63.
26. Brunnhuber K, Hill SJ, Ryan RE, Woodcock J (2010) Multimorbidity connections: laying the conceptual groundwork for evidence-based and patient-centred care. [Submitted to *BMC Family Practice*.]
27. Ryan R, Hill S (2010) Multimorbidity and communication with consumers. Invited paper presented by R Ryan. *National Medicines Symposium*, 26–28 May 2010, Melbourne.
28. Coulter A, Ellins J (2006) *Patient-Focused Interventions: A Review of the Evidence*. The Health Foundation, London.
29. Davis K, Stremikis K, Schoen C, et al. (2009) *Front and Center: Ensuring That Health Reform Puts People First*. Available from: http://www.commonwealthfund.org/. Accessed: 13 July 2009.
30. Schoen C, Osborn R, Huynh P, et al. (2005) Taking the pulse of health care systems: experiences of patients with health problems in six countries. *Health Affairs – Web Exclusive*, W5–509.
31. Tarn DM, Heritage J, Paterniti DA, Hays RD, Kravitz RL, Wenger NS (2006) Physician communication when prescribing new medications. *Archives of Internal Medicine* **166**, 1855–1862.
32. Fung CH, Setodji CM, Kung FY, et al. (2008) The relationship between multimorbidity and patients' ratings of communication constance. *Journal of General Internal Medicine* **23**, 788–793.
33. Jowsey T, Jeon YH, Dugdale P, Glasgow NJ, Kljakovic M, Usherwood T (2009) Challenges for co-morbid chronic illness care and policy in Australia: a qualitative study. *Australia and New Zealand Health Policy* **6**, 22.
34. Soubhi H, Bayliss EA, Fortin M, et al. (2010) Learning and caring in communities of practice: using relationships and collective learning to improve primary care for patients with multimorbidity. *Annals of Family Medicine* **8**, 170–177.
35. NHS (Scotland) (2005) *National Framework for Service Change in the NHS in Scotland: Self-Care, Carers, Volunteering and the Voluntary Sector: Towards a More Collaborative Approach*. Department of Health, UK. Available from: http://www.sehd.scot.nhs.uk/NationalFramework/Documents/electivecare/Selfcare230505.pdf. Accessed: 17 December 2008.
36. Manias E, Claydon-Platt K, McColl GJ, Bucknall TK, Brand CA (2007) Managing complex medication regimens: perspectives of consumers with osteoarthritis and healthcare professionals. *Annals of Pharmacotherapy* **41**, 764–771.
37. Ryan R, Hill S (2009) Multimorbidity decision burden for medicines not recognised. Letter 19 August 2009. *British Medical Journal* **339**, doi: 10.1136/bmj.b2803.

38. Easton K, Morgan T, Williamson M (2009) *Medication Safety in the Community: A Review of the Literature*. National Prescribing Service, Sydney. Available from: http://www.nps.org.au/research_and_evaluation/current_research/medication_safety_community. Accessed: 7 October 2010.
39. Ryan R, Santesso N, Hill S, Lowe D, Kaufman C, Grimshaw J (2011) Consumer-oriented interventions for evidence-based prescribing and medicines use: an overview of systematic reviews. *Cochrane Database of Systematic Reviews*, CD007768.

CHAPTER 15

Partners in care – an evidence-informed approach to improving communication with women in a hospital setting

Sophie Hill[1], *Maureen Johnson*[2] *and Mary Draper*[3]

[1]Coordinating Editor/Head, Cochrane Consumers and Communication Review Group, Centre for Health Communication and Participation, Australian Institute for Primary Care and Ageing, La Trobe University, Bundoora, Victoria, Australia

[2]Manager, Women's Consumer Health Information, The Royal Women's Hospital, Parkville, Victoria, Australia

[3]Independent Healthcare Consultant, Victoria, Australia

A continuous and explicit focus on quality improvement has become an important part of hospital activity in recent decades [1]. Research findings are integral to quality improvement, because new research may bring to light an innovative approach worth implementing or provide evidence that an existing approach should be stopped or restricted [2]. Change processes themselves have also become the subject of health services research – contributing to a better understanding of more effective ways to change complex organisational, professional or consumer behaviour – in the pursuit of more responsive healthcare and improved health outcomes.

This chapter contributes to this growing literature by examining how research on communication was integrated into a service improvement project at a major women's hospital in Victoria, Australia. We consider three issues associated with complex innovation and change processes: (1) what are the challenges associated with communication in hospitals, (2) what challenges do communication interventions present in seeking

The Knowledgeable Patient: Communication and Participation in Health – A Cochrane Handbook, First Edition. Edited by Sophie Hill.

evidence-informed healthcare and (3) what can we learn from different types of research to guide the selection of an intervention and inform the process of health service improvement?

Communication in hospitals is challenging

Good communication – affecting people's interactions and participation in all facets of the hospital experience – is challenging to all parties. There are many reasons why. People (patients, carers and health professionals) have individual preferences, behaviours and attitudes; speak different languages; and are influenced by a range of life experiences and cultures. Communication will always be affected by the social and cultural interplay between patients and clinicians. With the increasing complexity of the healthcare system, the knowledge or health literacy required to be a skilled patient or skilled carer is often high (see Chapter 16). There are barriers to communication, which perhaps get taken for granted, even simple ones. For instance, many patients have poor eyesight and hearing, which may make communication more difficult.

The context or institutional setting for health communication creates complexity. There are many clinical decisions that have to be taken in situations that are urgent or uncertain. Hospitals treat a significant number of patients each year for shorter lengths of stay. There are many demands on hospitals and constrained resources. There is also an organisational cultural issue about where resources are allocated. Some hospitals, and their health professionals, are yet to be convinced that an evidence-informed approach to communication will improve health outcomes or the patient's experience.

Communication is a quality and safety issue

Communication issues are a major component of patient-centred care [3], as feedback from consumers and family members about hospital experiences indicates. Communication is a key component of patient satisfaction surveys and may inform policies for achieving more responsive services internationally (see Chapters 1 and 2). But more than that, in a hospital and healthcare context, communication is a quality and safety issue. Poor communication can lead to adverse outcomes. For instance, poor communication between health professionals and patients and/or their families was a factor in a number of sentinel events recorded by the sentinel event program of the Department of Human Services, Victoria, Australia [4]. Poor communication is also a focus of many health service complaints [5, 6], and patients report that they do not always receive instructions about symptoms to watch out for when they are discharged from hospital [7]. Improving communication with patients on specific issues such as attending hospital for surgery may lead to more efficient use of resources [8].

Consumers have said that communication is a process of exchange – not just a process where health professionals inform or tell consumers what to do or what is happening [9]. The multidirectional nature of communication needs to be acknowledged so that effective communication can happen (see Chapter 2).

It is also important to understand the context for improving communication. At an individual level, good communication is embedded in relationships, with information sharing and decision-making happening over time and with all parties becoming more skilled over time. At an organisational level, good communication must be supported by institutional support, systems, resources, policies and education because individual consumers will encounter many hospital staff in any one episode of care.

Model for effective implementation of change – and communication

The conceptual framework for the project was based on the work by Richard Grol and Michel Wensing, outlined in their 2005 book (with co-editor Martin Eccles) titled *Improving Patient Care: The Implementation of Change in Clinical Practice*.

The main elements of the model are [10]:

1. Feed research findings or identified problems into a proposal for change.
2. Use a systematic and planned approach.
3. Formulate a concrete, well-developed and achievable proposal with clear targets. This encompasses the intervention, innovation or specific change that is the object of the change process.
4. Analyse and understand the target group – the setting, the people and what could hinder or promote a process of change.
5. Develop strategies for change, including strategies at all stages: dissemination, implementation and maintenance of the change.
6. Have an implementation plan with activities, tasks and timelines.
7. Evaluate and revise if necessary, and monitor using indicators.

We applied this model to an evidence-informed approach to quality improvement to communication in a hospital setting.

Researching quality improvement in a women's hospital

The Royal Women's Hospital in Melbourne is a tertiary referral centre that provides specialist health services for women and premature babies. In 2004 it was offered the opportunity to participate in a quality improvement project in collaboration with the Cochrane Consumers and

Communication Review Group and funded by the Victorian Quality Council [11, 12].

The hospital established a reference group with members from its Clinical Practice Improvement and Quality and Safety Units, senior clinicians, Consumer Liaison, Women's Consumer Health Information, and the Cochrane Consumers and Communication Review Group at La Trobe University in Melbourne.

The guiding philosophy was that purposeful health communication in hospitals, based on evidence, could improve health outcomes. Health communication is one of the most frequently performed 'interventions' in a hospital setting although it is not usually thought of this way. But if communication is conceived as tasks or interventions which are purposeful, planned and coordinated (see Chapter 3), it helps to map and delineate the various aspects of communication and the parties involved. This in turn is important for a quality improvement process, guided by the model described above.

Diagnostic analysis and prioritising an issue

The reference group discussed a range of communication issues. Criteria were developed to guide the choice of issue and included the amount and quality of data on the problem; its relation to quality, safety and organisational goals; staff readiness; resources for change; and consideration of organisational barriers and facilitators.

The group decided that women's decision-making about vaginal birth after Caesarean (VBAC) would benefit from the project and was an area for quality improvement.

The hospital's Caesarean rate was increasing, and whilst this mirrored national trends, emerging evidence on risks – particularly for women with later pregnancies – had encouraged clinical staff to consider strategies to ensure that Caesareans were performed appropriately and not unnecessarily. One of the strategies to reduce rates is to support the option of VBAC. Data on VBAC rates at the hospital, compared with some other Australian hospitals, showed that the hospital could aim to increase its support for VBAC.

Evidence to guide the quality improvement process

The next task was assembling and assessing the bodies of evidence or research findings to guide decisions. This included the clinical evidence on the effectiveness of different options for childbirth after a previous Caesarean, evidence on the effectiveness of communication interventions for decision-making about options for childbirth, research into consumers' preferences for decision-making styles and qualitative research findings to inform the intervention content and implementation process.

This chapter focuses mainly on issues associated with evidence-informed communication. However, the clinical evidence was a critical factor because the evidence for repeat Caesarean versus attempting VBAC had some uncertainty. Added to this was a variation in clinicians' opinion and preference. So women's preferences and values were even more important than for decisions where the evidence is strong and decision-making straightforward. The quality improvement goal was to ensure that women were provided with consistent, balanced, unbiased information about their options, so that shared decision-making between women and their doctors would lead to informed decisions, or at least decisions consistent with women's preferences and values.

The reference group looked at the evidence about clinical care and communication. This helped to establish what information was to be communicated to women, understand how current practice related to the evidence and analyse if there were barriers to change. Examining the evidence also allowed the reference group to develop a framework for communicating with women about VBAC and decide how the change would be evaluated.

Qualitative research – asking women patients and doctors in the hospital about decision-making processes – was done to inform the implementation stage, as it led to a better understanding of current practice, barriers and enablers to change.

Mapping the communication issue

Mapping the details and interactions involved in the communication or participation issue was an important step to prepare for searching for evidence related to communication interventions and for identifying potential solutions. In addition, it provided a better understanding of the organisational context. Communication and the diverse interactions that take place in a healthcare setting are complex. Addressing problems in the communication pathway requires a systematic approach to unpacking and mapping this complexity.

Mapping the communication problem was an iterative process. It was still part of the diagnostic phase (trying to isolate the range of problems), but a step towards identifying possible solutions [13]. The map also aided later decisions on what data to extract from trials, so that data were extracted consistently. It helped to unpack different aspects of communication and communication interventions. The categories for the map were:

- *context* for the issue, setting and people involved;
- *purpose* of interventions and relationship to quality improvement;
- *main parties* and *directions* of communication;
- intervention *features* and whether they are simple or complex;
- intervention *content*;
- *format*;
- *delivery* and *timing*.

However, the process of selecting possible solutions and tailoring them to the setting is a more complex process than applying the information from trials alone, and was informed by other research findings and discussion, as outlined below.

Searching for studies

One of the principles of evidence-informed quality improvement is that decisions for change should be founded on valid and reliable sources of information. This includes appropriate types of research addressing the range of questions posed and by discussion and consensus amongst key parties involved. Different questions are addressed by different forms of research:

What interventions are known to work?

This was informed by evidence from systematic reviews of controlled trials of communication interventions and influenced the choice of intervention.

What are people's views and experiences?

This was informed by evidence from reviews of qualitative studies and from single high-quality qualitative studies.

How should the intervention be implemented?

This was informed by quality improvement research in similar settings and consensus decision-making involving major parties concerned.

These principles guided the next stage of the project: searching for studies on communication interventions and issues associated with implementation. It was also crucial that the selection of studies was guided by the strength or quality of evidence and its relevance to the quality improvement question.

Assembling research to guide quality improvement

Evidence was assembled according to the questions and stages of the improvement process. Key research outputs are discussed below.

Evidence from systematic review of trials of decision aid intervention

There was strong evidence that a decision aid, when compared with usual care (i.e. no decision aid), produced better health outcomes and this guided the choice of a possible solution. Decision aids are increasingly used as a communication tool to assist doctors and patients in preference-sensitive situations. There are various formats and media, including pamphlets and video. Quality decision aids should have a number of components, including a description of – and the evidence for – treatment options, information to help people understand the options and to help them consider the personal importance of possible benefits and harms. They are a tool to help people participate in decision-making (for a major resource on decision aids, see the Ottawa Hospital Research Institute site, http://decisionaid.ohri.ca).

A Cochrane systematic review [14] of 34 trials of decision aids found that they are better than usual care in terms of the following outcomes: knowledge; decisional conflict and indecision; realism of expectations; and active involvement in decision-making. Decision aids decrease the rate of some major surgery. By 2009, this review was updated and included 55 controlled trials, with the earlier results confirmed [15].

Review of research of preferences and decision-making styles

A review of studies of women's preferences for childbirth options after Caesarean highlighted that women's decision-making incorporates personal as well as clinical factors [16]. For instance, women may opt for VBAC because of family obligations or the need for a shorter recovery.

A systematic review by Ronald Epstein, Brian Alper and Timothy Quill, physicians interested in improving discussion with patients about risks, recommended five important steps for shared decision-making and this information guided discussion about implementation of a decision aid. These steps are important in situations where doctors have to exercise clinical judgement, when women may have strong preferences and where the evidence base has some uncertainty [17]. This led to five key communication steps:

Step 1: Ask and understand about the woman's experiences, knowledge and expectations.
Step 2: Build partnerships by acknowledging complexity or difficulty of the issue.
Step 3: Provide evidence, but with a balanced discussion of the uncertainties.
Step 4: Present recommendations after integrating the doctor's clinical evidence with the woman's values and preferences.
Step 5: Check for understanding and agreement.

Using research to inform the content of the intervention

From relevant research, various topics were identified that women wanted covered in information materials. This helped in the design of the decision aid [18, 19]. Topics included the specific risks and benefits of vaginal and Caesarean birth, the evidence base of practical information about pain relief and interventions, the options for pain relief in labour and warning signs to be aware of in labour. Women also wanted information on the philosophy and policies of the hospital and staff, strategies to improve chances of a successful VBAC and the probability of success with specific caregivers.

Qualitative research to aid the change process

Qualitative research was undertaken with clinicians and with women to explore current practices and understand where and how communications interventions would be most effective. The interviews identified a number of issues critical to the effective implementation of improved communication with women.

A lack of understanding and compliance with existing practice regarding communication with women can be a challenge when implementing a new communication intervention. For the intervention to be successful there must be a commitment from medical staff to embrace an evidence-based approach to improved communication.

The interviews also raised issues related to the personal nature of the decision. For instance, women's confidence in a decision can be undermined by inconsistent advice from medical professionals, and when woman have made up their minds about VBAC, literature about risk may be less important to them than being supported with their decision.

Consistency of professional carer is of great importance to doctors and some patients, but consistency of care (hospital approach, opinion or advice) may be of greater importance to patients than getting to see the same doctor at each visit. As the research indicates, women liked to receive information from a variety of sources, and in addition to the evidence, women and doctors felt that information should be made available at different times throughout their care (particularly around the time of the primary Caesarean).

Finally, it was important that information materials for women were coordinated with organisational support for clinical guidelines or protocols [20, 21].

Once the research findings had been discussed, the implications needed to be translated into the actual business of the hospital. Information opportunities for women were noted, and they included points of discharge, antenatal education classes, consultations with doctors and support groups. Resources included the development of a decision aid, called 'Birth Choices: What Is Best for You?'

The five steps for shared decision-making were integrated into clinical practice guideline, the obstetric tool, and promoted more broadly.

Insights from the research stages of the project

The role of evidence of effectiveness

The project raised awareness that there is an evidence base for communication and shared decision-making interventions. A thorough literature review can highlight evidence gaps. As in other areas of evidence-based healthcare, the evidence base is evolving. Finally, if rigorous evidence of effectiveness on specific interventions or implementation strategies is not available from the published literature, descriptive studies provide a starting place for reviewing what is happening in other services.

The role of research on patients' experiences and views

The systematic identification of research findings on patients' or carers' experiences and the effects of interventions are complementary. Descriptive and qualitative research may provide information on issues such as cultural complexity, barriers and facilitators associated with particular strategies or information on people's preferences and views. The integration of findings from different types of research aids the process of selecting interventions and examining how to implement change.

Insights from the quality improvement stages of the project

Challenges to evidence-informed communication change processes

No matter how firmly based on evidence, implementation of quality improvement in hospitals is still a complex social process, involving many groups and individuals. Communication interventions are not instituted in a vacuum, but in a series of relationships, where the people move on, people's views change over time and there is variation in the clinical context. This means that measuring success is difficult.

Second, the intervention is being applied in an institutional context. This may mean that the intervention is applied inconsistently and there may be differing levels of support or commitment.

Benefits of evidence-informed communication change processes

An evidence-informed approach may strengthen the legitimacy of the project, however, and provides a way of managing risk. Understanding what evidence is available on effectiveness may lead to refining project objectives, making implementation more feasible and manageable.

Evidence cannot be taken 'off the shelf', but it should be examined and analysed in terms of its local application and relevance. It can ensure that a consistent and balanced approach is taken to informing all patients or carers. In the longer term, more research is needed to develop effective solutions tailored to contexts and people and which fit well into complex systems [22].

Despite the early view that this would be a fairly discrete area for a communication intervention, the choice of VBAC was anything but simple, the originally anticipated outcomes not straightforward and the project encountered all the challenges that face any quality improvement activity aimed at implementing evidence. VBAC is a contested area from both clinical and consumer viewpoints.

Some important outcomes were (1) demonstrating that there was a role for evidence in improving communication with consumers, (2) the ongoing role of evidence in developing consumer health information and strategies for improving health literacy, (3) the development of a decision aid on VBAC as part of the resources made available to women and (4) incorporation of consumer communication steps within the Clinical Practice Guideline.

References

1. Berwick DM (1989) Continuous improvement as an ideal in health care. *The New England Journal of Medicine* **320**, 53–56.
2. Grol R (2005) Introduction. In: Grol R, Wensing M, Eccles M, (eds.) *Improving Patient Care: The Implementation of Change in Clinical Practice.* Elsevier Butterworth Heinemann, Edinburgh, pp. 1–3.
3. Picker Institute Europe (2009) *Core Domains for Measuring Inpatients' Experience of Care.* Picker Institute Europe, Oxford.
4. Department of Human Services (DHS) Victoria (2005) *Sentinel Event Program Annual Report 2004–05.* Rural and Regional Health and Aged Care Service Division, Melbourne.
5. Office of the Health Services Commissioner Victoria (2005) *2005 Annual Report: One for All.* Office of the Health Services Commissioner, Melbourne.
6. Royal Women's Hospital (2005) *Quality of Care Report.* Royal Women's Hospital, Melbourne.
7. Schoen C, Osborn R, Huynh P, et al. (2005) Taking the pulse of health care systems: experiences of patients with health problems in six countries. *Health Affairs – Web Exclusive,* W5-509–W5-525.
8. Schofield W, Rubin G, Piza M, et al. (2005) Cancellation of operations on the day of intended surgery at a major Australian referral hospital. *Medical Journal of Australia* **182**, 612–615.
9. Draper M, Hill S (1996) *The Role of Patient Satisfaction Surveys in a National Approach to Hospital Quality Management.* Australian Government Publishing Service, Canberra. Available from: www.healthissuescentre.org.au/documents/ detail.chtml?filename_num=226730. Accessed: 12 January 2010.
10. Grol R, Wensing M (2005) Chapter 3. Effective implementation: a model. In: Grol R, Wensing M, Eccles M, (eds.) *Improving Patient Care: The Implementation of Change in Clinical Practice.* Elsevier, Butterworth Heinemann, Edinburgh, pp. 41–57.
11. Victorian Quality Council (VQC) (2007) *Communicating With Consumers and Carers – Part 1 – Pilot of Evidence-Based Selection of Communication Strategies to Improve Communication Between Consumers/Carers and Health Services.* VQC, Melbourne. Available from: http://www.health.vic.gov.au/qualitycouncil/activities/consumers.htm. Accessed: 25 October 2010.
12. Victorian Quality Council (VQC) (2007) *Communicating With Consumers and Carers – Part 2 – A Guide for an Evidence-Informed Approach to Improving Communication and Participation in Health Care.* VQC, Melbourne. Available from: http://www.health.vic.gov.au/qualitycouncil/activities/consumers.htm. Accessed: 25 October 2010.
13. Ovretveit J (1999) A team quality improvement sequence for complex problems. *Quality Health Care* **8**, 239–246.
14. O'Connor AM, Stacey D, Entwistle V, et al. (2003) Decision aids for people facing health treatment or screening decisions. *Cochrane Database of Systematic Reviews,* CD001431.

15. O'Connor AM, Bennett CL, Stacey D, et al. (2009) Decision aids for people facing health treatment or screening decisions. *Cochrane Database of Systematic Reviews*, CD001431.
16. Eden KB, Hashima JN, Osterweil P, Nygren P, Guise JM (2004) Childbirth preferences after cesarean birth: a review of the evidence. *Birth* **31**, 49–60.
17. Epstein RM, Alper BS, Quill TE (2004) Communicating evidence for participatory decision making. *Journal of the American Medical Association* **291**, 2359–2366.
18. Horey D, Weaver J, Russell H (2004) Information for pregnant women about caesarean birth. *Cochrane Database of Systematic Reviews*, CD003858.
19. Saisto T, Salmela-Aro K, Nurmi JE, Kononen T, Halmesmaki E (2001) A randomized controlled trial of intervention in fear of childbirth. *Obstetrics & Gynecology* **98**, 820–826.
20. O'Cathain A, Walters SJ, Nicholl JP, Thomas KJ, Kirkham M (2002) Use of evidence based leaflets to promote informed choice in maternity care: randomised controlled trial in everyday practice. *British Medical Journal* **324**, 643.
21. Stapleton H, Kirkham M, Thomas G (2002) Qualitative study of evidence based leaflets in maternity care. *British Medical Journal* **324**, 639.
22. Lavis JN, Davies HT, Gruen RL, Walshe K, Farquhar CM (2006) Working within and beyond the Cochrane Collaboration to make systematic reviews more useful to healthcare managers and policy makers. *Healthcare Policy* **1**, 21–33.

CHAPTER 16

Building health-literate societies

Sophie Hill[1], *Dianne B. Lowe*[2], *Chaojie Liu*[3] *and Nancy Santesso*[4]

[1]Coordinating Editor/Head, Cochrane Consumers and Communication Review Group, Centre for Health Communication and Participation, Australian Institute for Primary Care and Ageing, La Trobe University, Bundoora, Victoria, Australia

[2]Research Officer, Cochrane Consumers and Communication Review Group, Centre for Health Communication and Participation, Australian Institute for Primary Care and Ageing, La Trobe University, Bundoora, Victoria, Australia

[3]School of Public Health, La Trobe University, Bundoora, Victoria, Australia

[4]Department of Clinical Epidemiology and Biostatistics, McMaster University, Hamilton, Canada

Setting the scene

Health literacy has become a global health policy issue and is a concept critical to improving health outcomes. This chapter describes the health literacy concept and shows why it is relevant to health policy and practice. It proposes a conceptual approach to build the bridges between the health literacy concept, evidence-informed health communication and participation, and supportive and enabling strategies. It describes four areas of initiative internationally, which advance ideas and practices for how it can be built in individuals and societies.

Typically, people are living longer and with more than one health condition. At the same time, services are being provided with greater emphasis on self-management, minimally invasive procedures, shorter periods of hospital stay and earlier discharge. A consequence of this is that more information is required by individuals to manage their health or family's health in current service settings.

At the same time, information technology has expanded into our lives in such a way that, increasingly, computers and digital technologies are used for information, communication and entertainment. Technology has the potential to fill the health information demand described above, but this is not without its own set of problems (see Chapters 10 and 18). These

The Knowledgeable Patient: Communication and Participation in Health – A Cochrane Handbook, First Edition. Edited by Sophie Hill.

changes, forces and demands mean that individuals have to be *intelligent users* of services and information [1]. As consumers become more able to access information from an increasing array of sources, the skills of reading, writing and numeracy assume even greater importance [2].

The health literacy concept

At its simplest, health literacy is the ability to seek, find, understand and use health information [3]. Nutbeam [4] (drawing from work by Freebody and Luke, 1990) identifies three capacities, linked to what people can do, and combined with the concepts in this book, we provide the following outline:

1 *Functional health literacy* is the ability to read and write so that people can function in a health context. It is the result of education and health education. Health literacy also includes numeracy and relates to the capacity and confidence of people to understand and act on health statistics or information in numerical format.
2 *Communicative or interactive literacy* is to have the social and personal skills to apply information. Interactive literacy therefore builds on functional literacy and implies that people apply more complex cognitive, social and literacy skills to identify and use health information in communication with others, or apply or adapt it to changing circumstances. Applying and communicating information has increasingly come to mean consumers sharing and exchanging health experience and treatment information with each other and not just with health professionals [5].
3 *Critical health literacy* enables people to analyse information in a critical or reflective way. In turn, this gives them greater influence or control. In the language used in this book, this allows people to participate in different levels and with different roles (see Chapter 2), implying that organisations as well as individuals can be more or less literate, or more or less supportive of building health literacy. Critical literacy implies greater degrees of skills, expertise and motivation to navigate and use information in a critical sense.

Why is health literacy important?

Health literacy is therefore important to consumers' competence and ability to become active participants in their own health, health services and health systems in general [6]. This means that health literacy is important in thinking about actions at an individual level, but also actions at a service or societal level. Health literacy can be built, but the effects of poorer literacy have been the focus of much of the research so far. The consequences can be seen at the levels of individuals, health services and societies, and whilst this separation is a false one (because the consequences at one level impact on another), it helps to illustrate cascading effects and may also help to tease out where actions should be targeted.

Individual health impacts

The USA Office of Disease Prevention and Health Promotion states that poorer health literacy affects disease prevention behaviour and personal health management [7]. It can lead to reduced abilities around screening, child health management (diagnosis and medicine management) and following discharge instructions [8]. People with lower functional literacy are less likely to understand their medical conditions and choices [9].

Consequences on health services

It is not surprising that when we build up a picture, drawing from what is happening with individuals, we can observe that costs will grow and impacts spread. Research on healthcare utilisation patterns provides the challenging statistics that people with poorer health literacy seek care or enter the health system when they are sicker, they have a higher rate of hospital and emergency department use, and they may have admissions which are preventable [7].

Poorer health literacy is linked to more adverse events. The Institute of Medicine estimates that there are 1.5 million adverse events, many of which are preventable, and which are due to consumers' using medicines inappropriately [10].

Societal costs

Eichler and colleagues have estimated the cost of 'limited health literacy' in a systematic review of observational studies and systematic reviews [11]. They estimate that the costs of limited health literacy add from 3% to 5% of total health costs per year or between $US143 and $US7798 per person per year.

In addition, health literacy has an equity dimension given the basis of literacy in education. People with limited health literacy are more likely to report their health as poor. They have poorer health outcomes [7, 8]. It also undermines their sense of worth and dignity [7].

How can we build health-literate consumers and carers?

The individual, health service and societal impacts of poor health literacy can be addressed as part of public policy and through a key focus of health system improvement [12]. There are several reasons for this. Health literacy has universal aspects, for instance, knowledge of healthcare entitlements. It should be part of a social inclusion agenda because of the link between literacy and educational achievement. It has the capacity to weaken or strengthen the health system. For consumers it has life-course relevance. For universities, health practitioners and health services, it has implications for the health workforce and health service delivery. For governments, it has implications for health system policies and budgets.

Conceptual roadmap for building health literacy

The conceptual roadmap [13] outlined below provides a guide to shaping the direction of future strategies. It draws together and builds on the work in Chapter 2 of this book on evidence-informed health communication and participation and the work of Australian academics Don Nutbeam in public health and John Alford in public sector management.

First, in Chapter 2, it was argued that strategies to empower consumers should be informed by scientific approaches (e.g. evidence-based healthcare and systematic reviews) and democratic participation (e.g. individual or civic involvement). The chapter concluded: 'Integrating scientific approaches with democratic participation leads to awareness that not only should recommended health treatments be based where possible on rigorous evidence of benefit, but that approaches to communicating with and involving people should also be based where possible on evidence of effectiveness. This is the basis of *evidence-informed communication and participation*'. Interventions for communication and participation, as defined in the various chapters in this book, are integral to thinking about health literacy. The consequences of poorer literacy give us a potent reason on equity and health system grounds to invest in building the evidence on which interventions are effective.

Second, Nutbeam has argued that health literacy can be perceived as an asset [14] (and not simply a deficit in consumers). If it is an asset, it can be fostered in individuals, but also fostered by establishing supportive systems, for example, mandated communication skills training for health professionals, and enabling strategies, for example, investment in interpreting and translation services.

Third, co-production is a concept developed for examining public sector service provision by Alford [15]. Co-production implies that people do not just receive services, they help to produce them. In health, we rely on people to behave in certain ways, for example, taking the prescribed medicine because they agreed upon the course of action after a discussion with their doctor, exploring preferences and considering the risks and benefits. Here, this concept is applied 'backwards' to mean that increasingly consumers rely on health professionals to behave in certain ways and together they work to improve health.

If we take these three concepts together – evidence-informed communication and participation, literacy as an asset and co-production – we can argue that literacy can be built not only by directing strategies to individual consumers (such as more health information provision) but also by directing interventions to the community level, health professionals and health organisations.

Critically, however, building informed and active consumers is also about adopting *enabling* strategies [1, 13]. What are enabling strategies? Potentially, these are a diverse range of strategies that target various players at different levels (e.g. individual consumers, health practitioners, organisations and community). They are strategies that are designed to build people's capacity to act and use information, not just be passive recipients of information. They are also strategies that present information in a way that 'scaffolds' the patient and limits the impact of their own health literacy deficits. For instance, taking a major focus of this book as a guide, interventions to build health literacy in finding and using evidence-based health information could include a mass media campaign [16] to promote awareness of *The Cochrane Library*; the development of a tool to help doctors talk about the evidence in Cochrane reviews with patients; and training and support to help community organisations embed and translate evidence from systematic reviews into their informational resources. Policies could also form around systems to create incentives for health services to promote active and informed consumers through incentive funding models, standards, indicators and targets [17]. This would ensure that services establish supportive models and also consider how to address specific forms of inequity.

Initiatives for building health literacy

We now turn our attention to some of the initiatives globally which are relevant to building health literacy. We present four separate, but related, health literacy developments. First, we summarise the evidence accumulating on effective interventions. Second, we examine the development of a research tool to measure an effective health consumer. Third, we discuss health literacy issues in China, and lastly, the chapter draws on submissions to an Australian health reform process to identify how different players want health literacy recognised and improved.

Systematic reviews of interventions to improve health literacy

Evidence-informed communication and participation is about considering strategies that have been shown to improve health and communication outcomes. Evidence-based decision-making has been defined by Gray as decisions based on a 'systematic appraisal of the best evidence available in the context of prevailing values and resources available' [18]. This definition brings into play the centrality of people's views and preferences as well the context for decisions taken at many levels. What can we learn, then, from systematic reviews of interventions which have the purpose of improving people's health literacy?

Three systematic reviews [19–21] of the effects of interventions to improve health for those with poorer literacy show some positive effects and also demonstrate the range of interventions directed mainly to individual consumers but also to health professionals, including:

- using simplified language in verbal transactions in person or by phone;
- making information pamphlets or resources easier or simpler to read and understand;
- using pictorial or interactive computer-based formats;
- educational sessions tailored to people with lower literacy with a range of different formats and content;
- educational sessions for health professionals to build skills to interact.

The Effective Consumer Scale and OMERACT

Revisiting Haynes' definition of evidence-based medicine from Chapter 2, he highlighted that it is a set of tools and resources. The concept of health literacy, therefore, can be seen to infuse and inform other attributes of evidence-based healthcare – in particular, tools to measure the outcomes of an intervention intended to improve health literacy or aspects of literacy.

For example, the concept of an empowered and active consumer is influencing new approaches to delivering healthcare. Consumers are being encouraged to participate actively in the healthcare system and in their own health management. To achieve this, consumers have to be *equipped* to manage. Health literacy underpins such equipping concepts, including shared decision-making and expert patients. To know that consumers have the skills and attributes to manage, to feel empowered, to be active – and that this has benefited their health – researchers have to be able to measure this concept, that is, to put the concept into action.

Using the OMERACT process (Outcome MEasures in RheumAtology Clinical Trials), researchers, health professionals and people with rheumatoid arthritis from around the world are working together to develop a scale to measure an 'effective musculoskeletal consumer'. They first asked the question: what skills do people with arthritis need to manage their health effectively [22–24]? Pulling this information together with the growing research in this area and a large survey, they found that effectiveness can be assessed by how a consumer uses health information, clarifies and weighs values and priorities, communicates with others, negotiates roles and takes control, and decides and acts [25]. The Effective Consumer Scale asks whether an individual has the skills to effectively manage their health and healthcare – basically the critical, communicative and functional health literacy skills. This scale is proving to be responsive in self-management interventions, and future work will explore its use with other strategies to equip people to manage their health [26]. Without a scale such as this, it would be difficult to measure the success of interventions to improve health literacy skills.

Health literacy initiatives in China: where do Chinese consumers get health information?

Health literacy is a preoccupation not only of developed countries but of developing countries too. We now turn to China and discuss the emergence of a more 'critically' literate health consumer.

Without a gate-keeping mechanism in the Chinese healthcare system, consumers enjoy absolute freedom to bypass primary care and seek medical attention from tertiary hospitals. This is believed to have exacerbated the rapid escalation of medical expenditure and contributed to the fragmentation of healthcare services in China.

In 2008, the Ministry of Health initiated a 'health literacy for all' project, aiming at empowering consumers to make better decisions on lifestyle choices and health resource use. The 2008–2010 plan covers 66 basic and functional health literacy elements [27].

However, great challenges lie ahead. The health literacy project has adopted a top-down approach, resembling the 'Patriotic Health Campaign' social movement of the 1950s [28]. As Wang has commented [28], although such an approach is able to transmit basic health information to millions of people quickly, it might be too unsophisticated to address the increasingly complex health issues, often associated with social, economic and environmental determinants, that require a more participatory and locally empowering approach.

There are inequalities in health and health literacy between people of different ages, genders and education levels, and between those in urban and rural areas of China [29, 30]. People seek health information from a variety of channels. While health workers attempt to maintain their authoritative status, poor provider–consumer communication has inevitably diverted consumers to other sources of information. A recent survey in an outpatient clinic found that more than 90% of health workers believed that patients should be offered more critical information by health services, whilst more than 60% of patients thought that such information should be obtained from public media (unpublished data). In recent years, television and the internet have become the most important resources for health information [31, 32], with more than half of Chinese people gaining their health knowledge from television [31]. China has the second largest online population in the world, with more than 210 million people having access to the internet [33].

As health information becomes so much more easily accessible, contradictory information drawn from different sources has often resulted in confusion. A multinational survey undertaken by Ipsos has revealed that more than 65% of Chinese people are keen to learn more about nutrition (ranked number 1), but 30% are confused by the inconsistent information from various channels (ranked number 2) [34]. Recently, the central government has published a new set of measures to regulate online operations and ensure the accurate presentation of health information [27].

A television channel dedicated explicitly to health education will soon be ready to broadcast nationwide.

Health literacy in the context of national health reform

Health policy makers – and health organisations more generally – are recognising the importance of health literacy. In Australia, in 2008–2009, the National Health and Hospitals Reform Commission [35] drafted principles for reform. Of the 15 principles, 7 arguably have a direct link to health literacy [12] (those bolded below).

Australia's National Health and Hospitals Reform Commission Principles

- **People and family centred**
- **Equity**
- **Shared responsibility**
- **Strengthening prevention and wellness**
- Comprehensive
- Value for money
- Providing for future generations
- Recognising broader environmental influences which shape our health
- **Taking the long-term view**
- **Safety and quality**
- Transparency and accountability
- **Public voice**
- A respectful and ethical system
- Responsible spending on health
- A culture of reflective improvement and innovation

A range of organisations made submissions to the commission during its lifespan, and some linked their recommendations to a goal of improving health literacy and thereby achieving a better health system and improved health outcomes. The Royal Australasian College of Physicians linked health literacy and the public voice principle: with engaged patients better able to make healthier choices, manage their health, be involved in decisions, with potential for cost savings [36]. Choice, a non-government consumer-focused organisation, argued that Australia had promoted financial literacy through educational programmes in schools, and similar approaches could be taken to health literacy. The National Breast and Ovarian Cancer Centre [37] emphasised their collaborative approach to improving health outcomes based on consumer participation at all levels. Evidence-based information should be available in an accessible and timely way, and communication skills should be a compulsory competency for health professionals. The private sector also saw the high value in health literacy, with Microsoft HealthVault arguing for consumers to be in control of their personal health data [38].

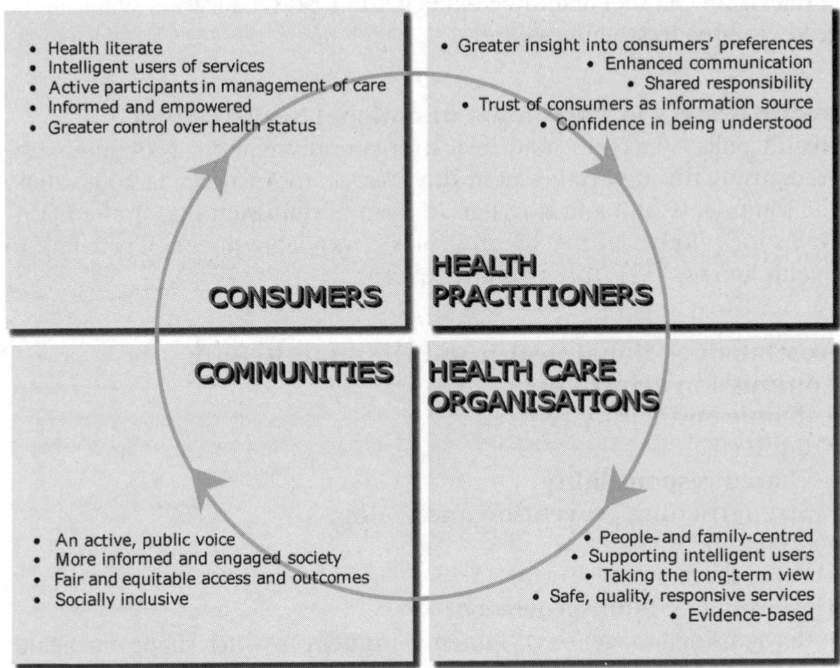

Figure 16.1 Building a health-literate society and envisaging the benefits.

Building a health-literate society: envisaging the benefits

Health literacy underpins actions at individual consumer, health practitioner, community and healthcare organisation levels. The benefits from improving health literacy are displayed in Figure 16.1.

Building health literacy, then, is not simply about providing consumers with more information. Information is a necessary part of a democracy, but we know from many reviews of the evidence that providing information alone does not lead to the kinds of health outcomes we seek. Health literacy is a cross-cutting policy issue that needs an evidence-informed approach that fosters capacity in individuals for people to work better with each other and for health systems and organisations to integrate health literacy concepts and strategies as a way to achieve a better health system and improved health outcomes.

References

1. Hill S, Draper M (2008) *Submission on the Public Health Voice principle to the National Health and Hospitals Reform Commission, Submission No. 403*. Australian National Health and Hospitals Reform Commission. Available from: http://www.health.

gov.au/internet/nhhrc/publishing.nsf/Content/403-hill-draper/$FILE/403%20-%20SUBMISSION%20-%20Sophie%20Hill%20and%20Mary%20Draper.pdf. Accessed: 20 December 2010.

2. Greenberg PB, Walker C, Buchbinder R (2006) Optimising communication between consumers and clinicians. *Medical Journal of Australia* **185**, 246–247.
3. Edwards M, Hill S, Edwards A (2009) Health literacy – achieving consumer 'empowerment' in health care decisions. In: Edwards A, Elwyn G, (eds.) *Shared Decision Making in Health Care: Achieving Evidence-Based Patient Choice*, 2nd ed. Oxford University Press, Oxford, pp. 101–107.
4. Nutbeam D (2000) Health literacy as a public health goal: a challenge for contemporary health education and communication strategies into the 21st century. *Health Promotion International* **15**, 259–267.
5. Fernandez-Luque L, Elahi N, Grajales FJ (2009) An analysis of personal medical information disclosed in YouTube videos created by patients with multiple sclerosis. *Studies in Health Technology and Informatics* **150**, 292–296.
6. Nutbeam D (2009) Defining and measuring health literacy: what can we learn from literacy studies? *International Journal of Public Health* **54**, 303–305.
7. US Department of Health and Human Services. *Fact Sheet: Heath Literacy and Health Outcomes*. Office of Disease Prevention and Health Promotion. Available from: http://www.health.gov/communication/literacy/quickguide/factsliteracy.pdf. Accessed: 20 December 2010.
8. Berkman ND, DeWalt DA, Pignone MP, et al. (2004) *Literacy and Health Outcomes. Summary, Evidence Report/Technology Assessment No. 87*. Agency for Healthcare Research and Quality, Rockville.
9. Schillinger D, Bindman A, Wang F, Stewart A, Piette J (2004) Functional health literacy and the quality of physician-patient communication among diabetes patients. *Patient Education and Counseling* **52**, 315–323.
10. Institute of Medicine (2010) *The Safe Use Initiative and Health Literacy: Workshop Summary*. The National Academies Press, Washington DC.
11. Eichler K, Wieser S, Brugger U (2009) The costs of limited health literacy: a systematic review. *International Journal of Public Health* **54**, 313–324.
12. Hill S (2008) *Improving Health Literacy: What Should – or Could – be on an Australian Policy Agenda?* Presentation to Department of Health and Ageing for the Cochrane Collaboration Policy Liaison Network, 12 November 2008, Canberra.
13. Hill S (2010) *Informed and Active Consumers: Building Health Literacy for Quality Use of Medicines* (Key Paper). National Medicines Policy Partnership Forum, 30 June 2010, Sydney.
14. Nutbeam D (2008) The evolving concept of health literacy. *Social Science & Medicine* **67**, 2072–2078.
15. Alford J (2009) *Engaging Public Sector Clients*. Palgrave Macmillan, Basingstoke.
16. Grilli R, Ramsay C, Minozzi S (2002) Mass media interventions: effects on health services utilisation. *Cochrane Database of Systematic Reviews*, CD000389.
17. Victorian Government (2009) *Doing It With Us Not for Us: Strategic Direction 2010–13*. Rural and Regional Health and Aged Care Services Division Victorian Government Department of Health, Melbourne. Available from: http://www.health.vic.gov.au/consumer/downloads/strategic_direction_2010-13.pdf. Accessed: 18 February 2010.
18. Gray JAM (2001) *Evidence-Based Healthcare: How to Make Health Policy and Management Decisions*. Churchill Livingstone, London, p. 12.

19. Pignone M, DeWalt DA, Sheridan S, Berkman N, Lohr KN (2005) Interventions to improve health outcomes for patients with low literacy. A systematic review. *Journal of General Internal Medicine* **20**, 185–192.
20. Coulter A, Ellins J (2007) Effectiveness of strategies for informing, educating, and involving patients. *British Medical Journal* **335**, 24–27.
21. Clement S, Ibrahim S, Crichton N, Wolf M, Rowlands G (2009) Complex interventions to improve the health of people with limited literacy: a systematic review. *Patient Education and Counseling* **75**, 340–351.
22. Tugwell PS, Wilson AJ, Brooks PM, et al. (2005) Attributes and skills of an effective musculoskeletal consumer. *The Journal of Rheumatology* **32**, 2257–2261.
23. Kirwan J, Heiberg T, Hewlett S, et al. (2003) Outcomes from the Patient Perspective Workshop at OMERACT 6. *The Journal of Rheumatology* **30**, 868–872.
24. Kirwan JR, Ahlmen M, de Wit M, et al. (2005) Progress since OMERACT 6 on including patient perspective in rheumatoid arthritis outcome assessment. *The Journal of Rheumatology* **32**, 2246–2249.
25. Kristjansson E, Tugwell PS, Wilson AJ, et al. (2007) Development of the effective musculoskeletal consumer scale. *The Journal of Rheumatology* **34**, 1392–1400.
26. Santesso N, Rader T, Wells GA, et al. (2009) Responsiveness of the Effective Consumer Scale (EC-17). *The Journal of Rheumatology* **36**, 2087–2091.
27. MOH (2009) Health literacy for Chinese citizens – essential knowledge and skills. *Chinese Health Education* **25**, 3–4.
28. Wang R (2000) Critical health literacy: a case study from China in schistosomiasis control. *Health Promotion International* **15**, 269–274.
29. Chen G, Ma L, Hu J, Chen Y, Xiao L, Tao M (2009) Comparison of health literacy between urban and rural. *Chinese Health Education* **25**, 163–166.
30. Xiao L, Ma L, Li Y, et al. (2009) Factors influencing health literacy of urban and rural Chinese. *Chinese Health Education* **25**, 323–326.
31. Mu J, Sun Q, Li Y (2004) Information channels of health literacy for an urban population in Danyang. *Chinese Journal of Rural Health Administration* **24**, 50–51.
32. Wang J (2006) Challenges facing health education and health promotion. *Chinese Primary Health Care* **20**, 65–66.
33. Long T (2008) Health education in an information era. *Applied Preventive Medicine* **14**, 31–33.
34. Life Time (2009) 65% Chinese are keen to learn more about nutrition. Life Time, cited by the Chinese Economic Network, Beijing. Available from: http://www.ce.cn/health/jkxw/hy/200904/27/t20090427_18924727.shtml. Accessed: 5 August 2009.
35. Australian Government (2009) *A Healthier Future for All Australians. Final Report of the National Health and Hospitals Reform Commission*. National Health and Hospitals Reform Commission, Canberra. Available from: www.nhhrc.org.au. Accessed: 12 December 2009.
36. Royal Australasian College of Physicians (2008) *Submission to the National Health and Hospitals Reform Commission, Submission No. 315*. Australian National Health and Hospitals Reform Commission. Available from: http://www.health.gov.au/internet/nhhrc/publishing.nsf/Content/315/$FILE/315%20-%20SUBMISSION%201%20-%20RACP-%20Principles%20for%20Australia%27s%20Health%20Care%20System.pdf. Accessed: 20 December 2010.
37. National Breast and Ovarian Cancer Centre (2008) *Submission to the National Health and Hospitals Reform Commission, Submission No. 122*. Australian National Health

and Hospitals Reform Commission. Available from: http://www.health.gov.au/internet/nhhrc/publishing.nsf/Content/122/$FILE/122%20National%20Breast%20and%20Ovarian%20Cancer%20Centre%20Submission.pdf. Accessed: 20 December 2010.

38. Microsoft Healthvault (2008) *Submission to the National Health and Hospitals Reform Commission, Submission No. 111*. Australian National Health and Hospitals Reform Commission. Available from: http://www.health.gov.au/internet/nhhrc/publishing.nsf/Content/111-mhv/$FILE/Submissions%20111%20-%20Microsoft%20Healthvault%20Submission.pdf. Accessed: 20 December 2010.

CHAPTER 17
Tools for building research capacity and knowledge transfer

Helen Dilkes[1], *Jessica Kaufman*[2] *and Sophie Hill*[3]
[1]Research Officer, Health Knowledge Network, Centre for Health Communication and Participation, Australian Institute for Primary Care and Ageing, La Trobe University, Bundoora, Victoria, Australia
[2]Research Officer, Cochrane Consumers and Communication Review Group, Centre for Health Communication and Participation, Australian Institute for Primary Care and Ageing, La Trobe University, Bundoora, Victoria, Australia
[3]Coordinating Editor/Head, Cochrane Consumers and Communication Review Group, Centre for Health Communication and Participation, Australian Institute for Primary Care and Ageing, La Trobe University, Bundoora, Victoria, Australia

Health services are increasingly involved in evaluating new models of care. This chapter describes the current literature on knowledge transfer and capacity building and the international initiatives putting these concepts into practice.

It then traces the history of a programme of support for hospitals undertaking rigorous research into consumer and carer participation. It explains the tools used to develop, understand, carry out and describe evaluative research. These tools include visual aids such as research maps and study design schematics, a conceptual framework for evaluation projects and multilevel research summaries.

The dynamic relationships of research, practice and policy

In order for research to influence policy and practice, it must be consumable: potential research users cannot apply research that they are unable to find or interpret. Research can be made accessible to users such as policy makers, health professionals and health consumers through capacity building and knowledge transfer.

The Knowledgeable Patient: Communication and Participation in Health – A Cochrane Handbook, First Edition.
Edited by Sophie Hill.

Capacity building

Capacity building is a term applied to healthcare strategies and processes which seek to create self-sustaining change in communities, individuals or organisations. Crisp and colleagues identify four approaches to capacity building: (1) policy changes within an organisation, (2) provision of skills to staff, (3) partnerships between groups or organisations and (4) community involvement initiatives. While Crisp et al. categorise these as distinct approaches, they acknowledge that in most cases a capacity-building strategy that causes change in one area (i.e. the policies of an organisation) will impact on other domains as well (i.e. the organisation's relationships with other groups) [1].

Several international initiatives to build research capacity have been taking place in recent years. The SUPPORT Project is an international collaboration of policy makers and scientists who aim to improve and increase the use of research evidence in policy decisions, particularly in low- to middle-income countries [2]. To this end, SUPPORT produces focused and accessible summaries of research, highlighting the features most relevant to policy and management. This is an example of a partnership approach to capacity building [1]: individual SUPPORT members from the science and policy sectors combine their knowledge to produce materials which in turn increase interaction and the flow of information between the larger research and policy communities. SUPPORT also develops resources to help users access evidence, commission and conduct reliable trials and apply resources effectively.

Practihc (Pragmatic Randomized Controlled Trials in Health Care) is a research and technology development network comprising researchers across 11 countries. The goal of Practihc is to increase the capacity of participating countries to evaluate their health systems, develop randomised controlled trials (RCTs) and promote international research and technology development cooperation [3]. Practihc provides tools, training and support for organisations and individuals, demonstrating the multilevel nature of capacity-building strategies.

Knowledge transfer

Knowledge transfer interventions are methods for making research information accessible and usable for a variety of audiences. Capacity building focuses on tools and training to build a user's ability to understand and utilise research; knowledge transfer initiatives seek the most accessible method for information delivery and develop strategies to enable stakeholders to put the knowledge into action [4]. While different countries and organisations use varying terms to describe and define knowledge transfer, the underlying principle is putting knowledge into action [5]. The Canadian Institutes of Health Research (CIHR), a primary funding organisation for Canadian health research initiatives, provides the following comprehensive definition of knowledge transfer (here referred to as 'knowledge translation'):

> Knowledge translation is the exchange, synthesis and ethically-sound application of knowledge – within a complex system of interactions among researchers and users – to accelerate the capture of the benefits of research for Canadians through improved health, more effective services and products, and a strengthened healthcare system [6].

The literature regarding knowledge transfer suggests that several features of an effort can influence its effectiveness. The information must be accessible and tailored to the intended audience, both in format and in language [7, 8]. The intervention should also be carried out according to a deliberate plan in order to reach the targeted individuals or groups [4]. Furthermore, the information should come from a trusted source [7].

Although knowledge transfer involves more than simple dissemination, getting information to the appropriate audience is a critical element of knowledge transfer initiatives. Lavis has identified the following two categories for information dissemination and application: *user-pull* efforts, directed towards making research and information available and accessible for users, and *producer-push* efforts, where researchers identify evidence of value to decision-makers and bring it to their attention [9]. Both *pull* and *push* efforts are based on the idea that research evidence is most likely to be put into action by target audiences that value evidence and are receptive to using it to inform their decisions [5].

There are many interventions for getting research from research producers to healthcare decision-makers in the health sphere, with most highlighting the importance of accessibility. A study conducted by Dobbins and colleagues, for example, indicates that community health organisation decision-makers prefer to receive brief 'bottom-line' bulletins describing research evidence in a short format with plain language [10].

To overcome the knowledge-to-action gap [4] and get research evidence into the hands of practitioners, policy makers and other potential research users, interventions must utilise capacity-building tools as well as knowledge transfer methods.

'The best way to learn is to teach': research users as research creators

One way to build capacity among research users is to transform them into research creators. When healthcare decision-makers seek to develop or improve interventions regarding consumer participation, they are encouraged to base their decisions on evidence from the field. This makes them research users. However, with support and assistance, they can implement their own evaluative studies of interventions. This not only enhances their knowledge and capacity for using research, but also expands the body of evidence available to other individuals and organisations.

In Australia, the Victorian Department of Health describes the process cycle by which healthcare organisations can both contribute to health participation research and continuously improve participation interventions [11]. The cycle begins with a development and planning stage, when the intervention is conceived or improved upon. This stage is followed by implementation, evaluation and monitoring, publishing and promoting, and learning from the evidence. The cycle repeats as new insight influences existing interventions or inspires new developments.

In 2007, the Department of Health – then the Department of Human Services – puts this cycle into practice with the Evaluating Effectiveness of Participation (EEP) projects.

Project background

The Cochrane Consumers and Communication Review Group (CC&CRG) was engaged by the Victorian Department of Human Services to support its EEP projects, conceived as a reflection of the newly launched Victorian health policy 'Doing it with us – not for us' [11]. The policy development process identified a lack of rigorous studies evaluating the effects of interventions for consumer participation, with an eye on quality and safety issues. Through the EEP projects, the Department of Human Services would fund health services to undertake evaluations of either a new and innovative or an existing consumer participation initiative.

Rigorous evaluation was encouraged so that project results might eventually qualify for (potential) inclusion in systematic reviews published by the Cochrane Effective Practice and Organisation of Care (EPOC) Group or the CC&CRG – the Cochrane groups most likely to publish reviews in this field. Participants were asked to develop their projects using one of the study designs accepted by the EPOC and CC&CRG: an RCT, a quasi-RCT, a controlled before-and-after (CBA) study or an interrupted time series (ITS) study.

In the past, consumer participation interventions were likely to be evaluated by process evaluations such as surveys of one site or case studies [12]. The CC&CRG promoted rigorous study designs for researching the effects of interventions in the EEP projects in order that the information gained from the EEP studies could contribute to an international evidence base around issues of communication and participation with a focus on consumers.

The CC&CRG was in a key position to provide support to the health services in their applications for funding and in subsequent project implementation. In addition to aiding the organisations involved in EEP projects, CC&CRG support and information could be fed back to the health sector as a whole via the group's knowledge transfer service – the

Health Knowledge Network – ensuring broad dissemination of knowledge. The project would also build research capacity for the health services, as research and policy interactions such as the collaboration between the CC&CRG and EEP health services could increase the use of research evidence by participating organisations [13].

The CBA study design – which all participating health services chose to attempt over RCTs or ITS studies – presented challenges for the practitioners, managers and others undertaking the research. Many of the health service researchers knew little about designing or carrying out a CBA study. They also expressed concern about finding a control site and dealing with complex statistical issues, so multidisciplinary teams were required at all sites. Projects were encouraged to seek personalised assistance relevant to evaluating consumer participation interventions from the CC&CRG.

Four Victorian health services, both rural and metropolitan, received funding for EEP projects. The focus of the four investigations is provided below by their project titles, as presented in funding submissions. This chapter focuses on the project undertaken by South West Healthcare, a large regional hospital in western Victoria.

Cobram District Hospital
Nursing home case management and family involvement in residents' care (a new model for encouraging family involvement)

Orbost Regional Health
New methods for engaging consumers in planning and development of health services (a new model for feedback from consumers/community)

Peter MacCallum Cancer Centre
Improving medication safety through consumer partnerships during transitions from home to hospital and back again (medication reconciliation processes)

South West Healthcare
The impact of consumer and carer delivery of training on clinician attitude, confidence and competence in working in partnership with consumers and families (consumer/family members' stories of mental health, in training of clinicians) [14]

The South West Healthcare project intended to focus on the effects of supplementing staff training with the personal stories of consumers and their family members regarding mental health. The project sought to determine the intervention's effects on clinician confidence, competence (self-reported) and attitudes.

All the projects were able to utilise assistance from the CC&CRG throughout the project's phases, including initial project conception, research implementation and report writing. This support comprised both visual and conceptual research aids, as well as personalised assistance with development of the research proposals.

Aids for research

Visualising healthcare

During project conception, researchers asked for advice on relevant study designs and specific study design issues, such as how to develop a research question; how to develop and describe interventions; and how to identify relevant outcomes for consumer participation, considering what is achievable with a CBA study design and with the EEP funding timeline in mind. The CC&CRG developed visual tools to respond to these requests.

Study design

People unfamiliar with research study design can experience challenges in devising, carrying out and analysing the results from studies. Evidence suggests that visual models or frames can clarify study design features and aid understanding [15]. For instance, Jackson and colleagues developed the graphic appraisal tool for epidemiological studies when they found that students were struggling to assess study quality. Their design helped students understand and critically appraise epidemiological studies [15].

The CC&CRG created diagrams illustrating RCTs and CBA study designs in order to clarify the study features for the EEP applicants [16]. South West Healthcare researchers chose to carry out a CBA study and referred to the diagram provided by the CC&CRG to develop their project (see Figure 17.1). This frame illustrates the timing or progress of activities during a CBA study: recruiting participants or establishing the intervention and control groups, measuring before the intervention is implemented, implementing the intervention and measuring after implementation of the intervention.

Research project map

This tool outlines the key issues to consider when undertaking a high-quality research project. Framing a research question helps to conceive of the project before you begin: the main focus of the study in terms of the interventions, participants and main outcomes of the study [17, 18]. The PICO structure then provides a clear framework for the detail of conducting and reporting on the research in terms of identifying *p*articipants to be included; developing the *i*ntervention to implement during the study (which may involve consumers assisting with its development through

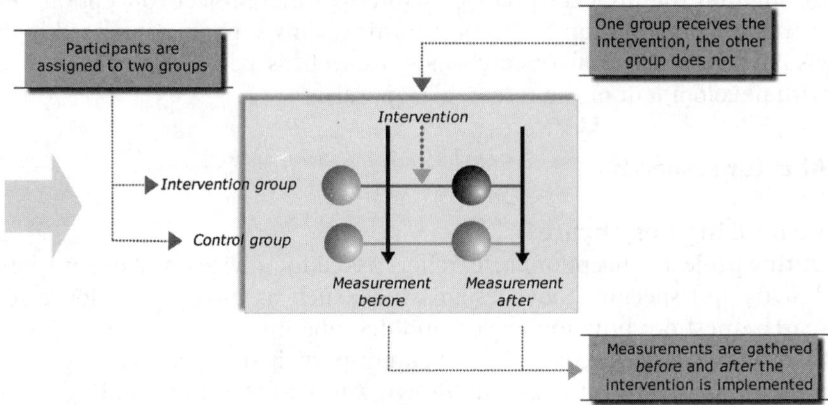

Figure 17.1 Diagram and descriptions of key aspects of a controlled before-and-after study design.

focus groups, for example); establishing a control group for *c*omparison; and selecting key *o*utcomes of interest.

The visual PICO map the CC&CRG provided for South West Healthcare showed examples from their own project, as they corresponded to the different elements of the PICO outline (see Figure 17.2). With this visual aid, researchers could confirm that their research was appropriately structured.

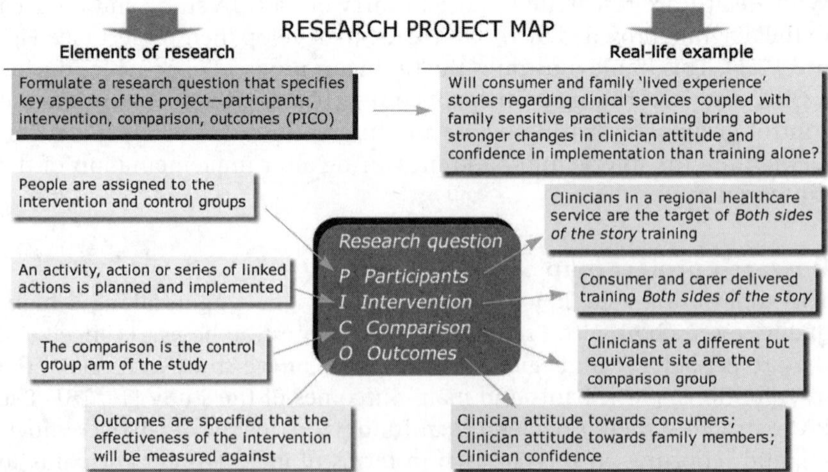

Figure 17.2 Map showing key elements of research, with examples from the South West Healthcare project undertaken in Victoria, Australia.

Conceptual framework

In addition to visual aids, the CC&CRG provided support in the form of a conceptual framework to help participants develop and implement their intervention evaluation projects.

The framework was included as an appendix to the Department of Human Services Expression of Interest document, provided to all potential applicants [19]. It is a brief outline supplying background information on consumer participation evaluation projects and answers key questions to help participants develop their submissions. Policy makers and non-researchers may have little experience conducting or analysing research, and this can lead to serious problems when decisions are based on biased or misinterpreted evidence [20]. A lack of understanding can also sour a person's attitude towards research, causing them to see evidence as too boring or complicated and less convincing than a gut feeling [20].

The EEP framework seeks to introduce research concepts in an accessible way, providing definitions of important terms such as 'consumer and carer participation' and 'intervention'. The framework can help health services identify quality and safety areas in need of improvement, potential programmes that could be improved by the project and new interventions that could be developed. The information in the framework also includes examples to clarify and categorise possible outcomes and effects, and directs researchers to *The Cochrane Library* for further resources and information.

Supersynthesis of research: knowledge transfer

EEP researchers required assistance with searches and search strategies, and requested that the CC&CRG identify applicable systematic reviews and studies. Finding appropriate and helpful systematic reviews is one of the primary obstacles to non-researchers using research evidence in policy- and decision-making [13]. To disseminate relevant information to the EEP research users, the CC&CRG created a knowledge transfer system, featuring carefully designed evidence bulletins. Later in the projects, participants wanted advice or a framework on report writing. Resource bulletins highlighted helpful resources in this area.

Evidence bulletins are accessible, multilevel research summaries that summarise Cochrane systematic reviews of evidence. A major challenge facing those who wish to use Cochrane systematic reviews for research is the complexity of the review language and format [21–23]. Evidence bulletins translate reviews into language that is simple, clear, brief and tailored for a non-expert audience [7].

Bulletins have a three-tiered structure that allows readers to quickly gather as much or as little detail as they need. According to Lavis, the most effective way to deliver information from systematic reviews is in a 1:3:25 'graded entry' format, with a 1 page take-home messages, a 3-page executive summary and a 25-page detailed report [23]. This allows readers to skim key messages to determine if the information is relevant to them before choosing whether to read in more detail. Evidence bulletins are 5 to 8 pages long and use an adapted 1:3:25 structure, shown in Figure 17.3. The first page is an overview of key messages, the middle pages feature a more detailed summary of the review and the final pages contain an evidence table which expresses complex technical information in a concise and standardised format [24].

Resource bulletins are 1-page e-bulletins that highlight local and international resources as needed by people in the field. One resource bulletin developed for the EEP participants included descriptions of and links to programmes such as the Trial Protocol Tool and the Clinical Trials Simulator. Both are online tools that help users design and test potential research trials [3].

These bulletins were created for the EEP projects initially, but are now shared with a broader audience, including healthcare professionals, consumers and policy makers. This wider initiative is now carried out by the Health Knowledge Network, which works in conjunction with the CC&CRG.

Project outcome

Projects were encouraged to focus on a few relevant outcomes during implementation in order to keep the evaluation to a manageable size and to enable focused and meaningful reporting. The South West Healthcare project focused on three primary outcomes and their findings are reported in relation to these [25].

Attitudes towards consumers

- Significant improvement in attitudes related to consumer perspective on recovery, hope for recovery, role in professional development and participation in treatment planning.
- Significant reduction in stigmatising attitudes.

Attitudes towards family members

- Significant improvement in clinician attitudes towards family members related to blame, empowering family members, routine family involvement in treatment and treatment planning, and ongoing role for family members in their professional development.

Clinician confidence

- Clinician confidence was significantly improved by training, but was not significantly enhanced by consumer and family participation in the training.

Participation in the EEP project not only provided South West Healthcare with important information regarding the outcomes of a new intervention, but also supplied those carrying out the research with the

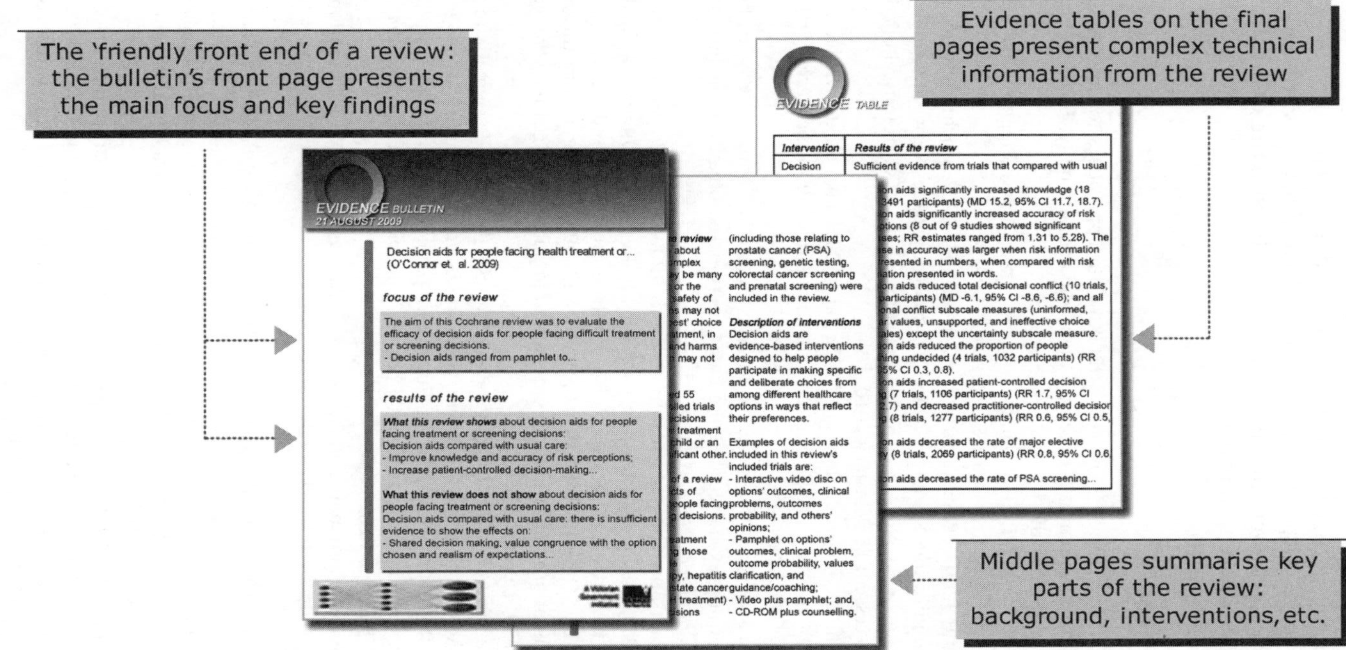

Figure 17.3 Diagram of an indicative evidence bulletin, showing three different levels of complexity of information.

skills and knowledge necessary to perform further research and potentially publish their results in the future, thus expanding the body of evidence surrounding consumer participation interventions.

In 2009, the Victorian Department of Health Services announced a second EEP programme for supporting research, with the CC&CRG assisting in the development of proposals.

References

1. Crisp B, Swerissen H, Duckett S (2000) Four approaches to capacity building in health: consequences for measurement and accountability. *Health Promotion International* **15**, 99–107.
2. SUPPORT website. Available from: http://www.support-collaboration.org/objectives.htm. Accessed: 18 December 2009.
3. Dilkes H (2007) *Resource Bulletin*, 12 December 2007. Cochrane Consumers and Communication Review Group, Health Knowledge Network. Available from: http://www.latrobe.edu.au/chcp/assets/downloads/HKN_resourcebulletin_121207.pdf. Accessed: 18 February 2010.
4. Graham ID, Logan J, Harrison MB, et al. (2006) Lost in knowledge translation: time for a map? *The Journal of Continuing Education in the Health Professions* **26**, 13–24.
5. Wilson MG, Lavis JN, Travers R, Rourke SB (2010) Community-based knowledge transfer and exchange: helping community-based organizations link research to action. *Implementation Science* **5**, 33.
6. Canadian Institutes of Health Research (2004) *Knowledge Translation Strategy 2004–2009*. Canadian Institutes of Health Research, Ottawa. Available from: http://www.cihr-irsc.gc.ca/e/26574.html#defining. Accessed: 10 May 2010.
7. Green LW, Ottoson JM, Garcia C, Hiatt RA (2009) Diffusion theory and knowledge dissemination, utilization, and integration in public health. *Annual Review of Public Health* **30**, 151–174.
8. Tugwell P, Robinson V, Grimshaw J, Santesso N (2006) Systematic reviews and knowledge translation. *Bulletin of the World Health Organization* **84**, 643–651.
9. Lavis JN (2006) Research, public policymaking, and knowledge-translation processes: Canadian efforts to build bridges. *The Journal of Continuing Education in the Health Professions* **26**, 37–45.
10. Dobbins M, Rosenbaum P, Plews N, Law M, Fysh A (2007) Information transfer: what do decision makers want and need from researchers? *Implementation Science* **2**, 20.
11. Victorian Government (2009) *Doing It With Us Not for Us: Strategic Direction 2010–13*. Rural and Regional Health and Aged Care Services Division Victorian Government Department of Health, Melbourne. Available from: http://www.health.vic.gov.au/consumer/downloads/strategic_direction_2010-13.pdf. Accessed: 18 February 2010.
12. Marjanovic S, Hanney S, Wooding S (2009) A historical reflection on research evaluation studies, their recurrent themes and challenges. *RAND Technical Report 2009*. Available from: http://www.rand.org/pubs/technical_reports/TR789/. Accessed: 18 February 2010.

13. Lavis JN (2009) How can we support the use of systematic reviews in policymaking? *Public Library of Science Medicine* **6**, e1000141.
14. Victorian Government (2008) *Findings of the Evaluating Effectiveness of Participation Projects*. Available from: http://www.health.vic.gov.au/consumer/conferences/findings.htm. Accessed: 18 February 2010.
15. Jackson R, Ameratunga S, Broad J, et al. (2006) The GATE frame: critical appraisal with pictures. *Evidence-Based Medicine* **11**, 35–38.
16. Ryan R, Hill S, Broclain D, Horey D, Oliver S, Prictor M (2009) *Study Design Guide*. Cochrane Consumers and Communication Review Group. Available from: http://www.latrobe.edu.au/chcp/assets/downloads/StudyDesignGuide110809.pdf. Accessed: 14 April 2010.
17. Cochrane Effective Practice and Organisation of Care Review Group (2002) *Data Collection Checklist*. Revised by Laura McAuley – with input from Craig Ramsay. Available from: http://epoc.cochrane.org/sites/epoc.cochrane.org/files/uploads/datacollectionchecklist.pdf. Accessed: 14 April 2010.
18. Higgins J, Green S (eds.) (2009) *Cochrane Handbook for Systematic Reviews of Interventions Version 5.0.2*. Available from: www.cochrane-handbook.org. Accessed: 14 April 2010.
19. Department of Human Services (2007) *Evaluating Effectiveness of Participation Projects*. Available from: http://www.health.vic.gov.au/consumer/downloads/evaluating_effectiveness_participation.pdf. Accessed: 18 February 2010.
20. Jewell CJ, Bero LA (2008) 'Developing good taste in evidence': facilitators of and hindrances to evidence-informed health policymaking in state government. *The Milbank Quarterly* **86**, 177–208.
21. Rosenbaum S, Glenton C, Cracknell J (2008) User experiences of evidence-based online resources for health professionals: user testing of The Cochrane Library. *BMC Medical Informatics and Decision Making* **8**, 34.
22. Rosenbaum S, Glenton C, Oxman A (2008) [O07-25] Summaries of evidence for health policymakers in low and middle income countries (LMIC). *16th Cochrane Colloquium*, Freiburg, 3–7 October 2008.
23. Lavis J, Davies H, Oxman A, Denis JL, Golden-Biddle K, Ferlie E (2005) Towards systematic reviews that inform health care management and policy-making. *Journal of Health Services Research & Policy* **10** (Suppl. 1), 35–48.
24. Ryan RE, Kaufman CA, Hill SJ (2009) Building blocks for meta-synthesis: data integration tables for summarising, mapping, and synthesising evidence on interventions for communicating with health consumers. *BMC Medical Research Methodology* **9**, 16.
25. Bateman J, Lyon E (2008) *Both Sides of the Story*, presentation at Department of Human Services Victoria, 15 September 2008. Available from: http://www.health.vic.gov.au/consumer/conferences/findings.htm. Accessed: 18 February 2010.

CHAPTER 18
Emerging technologies for health communication

Yannis Pappas[1] *and Josip Car*[2]
[1]Deputy Director, eHealth Unit, Department of Primary Care and Public Health, Faculty of Medicine, Imperial College London, London, United Kingdom
[2]Director, eHealth Unit, Department of Primary Care and Public Health, Faculty of Medicine, Imperial College London, London, United Kingdom

Introduction

This chapter has three objectives:

1 To introduce the reader to an array of health information technologies that may facilitate patient communication
2 To discuss the potential of these technologies to improve healthcare through improved communication and participation
3 To discuss the challenges of implementing communication technologies.

This is an issue because . . .

A consumer-oriented technology explosion has changed banking, education and telecommunications, and is now changing healthcare. The use of information communication technologies (ICTs) such as cell phones, personal digital assistants (PDAs) and iPods is widespread. The ubiquitous nature of ICTs and the ever-increasing availability of the internet is changing the way patients/consumers think about and, more importantly, seek healthcare. Today, people of all backgrounds use ICTs to access their own medical records through web portals, communicate online with others (on a personal basis or in virtual communities), transmit health data using the telephone or the web and surf the internet to find information about health and health services.

Both demand by consumers and initiative by health services and government have driven change [1, 2]. As a result, a new field for

The Knowledgeable Patient: Communication and Participation in Health – A Cochrane Handbook, First Edition.
Edited by Sophie Hill.

researching, planning and implementing ICTs in healthcare has emerged under the umbrella term eHealth. Because eHealth is in a state of flux, there is no single agreed definition. For the purposes of this chapter, we use Pagliari's 2005 adaptation of Eysenbach's [3] definition:

> eHealth is an emerging field of medical informatics, referring to the organisation and delivery of health services and information using the Internet and related technologies. In a broader sense, the term characterises not only a technical development, but also a new way of working, an attitude, and a commitment for networked, global thinking, to improve healthcare locally, regionally and worldwide by using information and communication technology [4].

In conjunction with developments in eHealth, models of healthcare delivery will have to evolve from being clinician driven to being patient centred, with a central aim to facilitate enhanced communication and patient participation in all stages of decision-making [5].

eHealth: range and relevance to patient communication

eHealth applications vary considerably, not only because they naturally adopt the characteristics of the several technological tools that underline their use, but also because they are dependent on the organisational, clinical, economic and psychosocial conditions in which they are used. In a world of rapidly developing IT solutions and continuously re-evaluated and re-structured healthcare systems, the attempt to produce a universally agreed map of eHealth applications seems an impossible venture. Notably, a 2005 systematic review by Oh and colleagues identified 41 unique definitions for eHealth [6]. Nevertheless, if we take an approach based on the types of services the various eHealth tools provide to consumers, the range of existing and emerging applications may be classified under three broad categories, as provided in Table 18.1.

Health information sharing and electronic health records

Effective implementation of eHealth is not, however, simply achieved through the mere existence of the tools. Sharing of clinical information is also essential to the future development of modern healthcare systems, which are increasingly characterised by the involvement of many specialist healthcare providers [8]. In most developed countries, patients now commonly receive their healthcare from a range of practitioners, many of whom work at different locations. For most people these include health centres, pharmacies, dentists, opticians, physiotherapists, complementary health therapy centres, dietitians and trainers, a

Table 18.1 eHealth services for healthcare consumers.

Service type	Description	Examples
Information provision	Electronic provision of health and wellness information	Health portals or information tools for consumers to retrieve or tailor health information Selection of information based on personal profile, disease or a particular need, such as travel or cross-border healthcare Example of portal: USA site 'Health Plus', http://www.healthplus-ny.org/en/index_ENG_HTML.html
Application interface for health management	Electronic interface between consumers and health service providers to better support consumers' use of health services	Electronic appointment booking, obtaining test results or ePrescriptions Example of portal: UK site 'NHS Choices', http://www.nhs.uk/Pages/HomePage.aspx
Homecare and telemedicine	Provision of care at the patient's personal environment outside traditional healthcare facilities	Pacemaker monitoring, remote ECG, dermatology, wound management Example of portal: Australian site 'Telemedcare', http://www.telemedcare.com.au/

Source: Derived from [7].

variety of hospitals and laboratory services and, occasionally, ambulance services.

Increasingly, self-monitoring and guided self-care is also used. The ideal in this respect is for professionals and also patients to have the ability to simultaneously access and seamlessly transfer, contribute to and integrate clinical data from disparate sources. The electronic health record (EHR) encompasses all health information regarding an individual and is the primary source for recording and documenting health data in several media forms [9]. The substantial international investment in EHRs and related eHealth applications is based on the premise that the development of accurate and readily accessible electronic patient records can improve the quality, safety and efficiency of healthcare. Also, many of the practical benefits of EHRs in improving quality of care, patient safety and public health may arise from the secondary use of data sets for health monitoring, planning and research. However, this gives rise to multiple ethical and technical challenges about access to and use of data. Also, relatively little is still known about public attitudes to secondary uses of such data.

How eHealth might affect the relationship between the patient and the healthcare system?

The use of eHealth could change the relationship between patients and health providers in more ways than one. The potential benefits are considerable and multidimensional. Claims of improved access, choice, communication and health outcomes abound in the literature [7, 10, 11]. Overall, there is evidence that various eHealth initiatives around the world have contributed to improving patient choice and access to a personalised healthcare [12–14], which can have a positive effect on patient outcomes and social care [15].

Anticipated benefits of eHealth

Improved patient access and choice

eHealth facilitates access to shared systems of care that enable the coordination of activities of all users, which often happens at distance. There is general consensus that consumers are becoming increasingly involved in, and wish to be more informed about, the medical decision process. As a result, provider–consumer interactions are no longer limited to the face-to-face consultation, but now make use of several media communication channels, such as email [16], mobile text messaging [17], telephone [18] and web-based communication applications [19]. Web-based health portals such as Google Health, Microsoft HealthVault and HealthSpace allow consumers and professionals to access, share and amend medical records and health-related information [20].

Enhanced communication between professionals

eHealth applications can be used to record and transfer details of the patient's health, to monitor patient progress and also to provide advice at a distance via the use of homecare and telemedicine interventions, such as teleradiology and telecardiology [20].

Improved health outcomes

Enhanced communication between healthcare professionals, as well as between professionals and consumers, is required for the treatment of the ageing population of developed societies, as well as for people with long-term conditions (e.g. diabetes and hypertension). It is possible that the successful use of EHRs, supported by the necessary organisational and social changes [21], may substantially reduce costs, improve efficiency [22] and enhance patient safety by reducing medical errors [23]. Tailored interventions have led to positive outcomes across a variety of interventions, such as binge drinking [24], nutrition and diet [25], and smoking [26].

A systematic review by Jimison and colleagues [27] reported that interactive consumer eHealth applications tended to have a positive effect on patient outcomes when they provided a complete feedback loop that included (a) monitoring of current patient status; (b) interpretation of these data in light of established, often individualised, treatment goals; (c) adjustment of the management plan as needed; (d) communication back to the patient with tailored recommendations or advice; and (e) repetition of this cycle at appropriate intervals. Systems that provided only one or a subset of these functions were less consistently effective.

Potential risks of using ICTs

We must not ignore the potential risks associated with the implementation of eHealth in complex environments such as healthcare services [23, 28, 29]. The introduction of various ICTs in healthcare, rightly intended to support and enhance communication and participation, inevitably affects associated aspects of care within the healthcare 'ecosystem' dramatically. These changes include interruptions to several aspects of work, such as clinical decision-making practices [30], patient pathways, workflow [31] and communication between participants [32]. For example, media such as the pager or telephone that are used for communication between healthcare professionals are highly interruptive, and can cause memory disruptions and lead to errors [33]. The same is also true of more complex applications such as computer decision support systems (CDSS), which can generate medical errors in the form of erroneous prescription recommendations [34].

Putting research into policy or practice will require . . .

There is evidence that eHealth interventions have the potential to shape healthcare systems that are fit for the twenty-first century [35]. Consequently, there have been many attempts to increase the use of eHealth in healthcare systems internationally. However, recent research suggests that poorly designed and inadequately evaluated eHealth interventions fail to integrate with healthcare systems and to deliver anticipated health outcomes and cost benefits [22, 36].

Because eHealth introduces a number of interruptive processes and changes to already complex healthcare systems, the development of a comprehensive agenda for research, planning and implementation is essential [37]. In doing so, three individual, but reasonably integrated, steps are crucial:

1 First, to construct a solid evidence base through sound original studies and appropriate synthesis of findings in rigorous systematic reviews that identify topic-specific and cross-cutting messages for safe, effective and cost-effective implementation of eHealth tools [38, 39]. Such an approach will contribute to a comprehensive evaluation and

understanding of factors that facilitate or hinder the successful use of eHealth tools and the range and magnitude of effects.

2 Second, to create a theoretical framework to understand change within a broader social and organisational context in order to understand the normalisation of activities and processes in eHealth (i.e. how they become part of everyday practice). eHealth initiatives are usually characterised by pilot implementations that cease when an individual project is over. eHealth has failed so far to become widely implemented because processes do not normalise easily [40, 41]. eHealth research, planning and implementation could benefit from an expansion in its use of methodological/theoretical models. A common methodological framework eases the communication process and assists researchers to build on each other's work. Currently, there is a distinct absence of such a scholarly approach in eHealth, and the lack of a common theoretical framework impedes interdisciplinary communication, interpretation and integration of findings.

3 Third, to involve multidisciplinary teams of specialists not only in research but also in decision-making, planning and implementation. This should focus not only on exploring the immediate contextual elements of eHealth (e.g. clinical and psychosocial impact), but also on developing a solid understanding of the organisational, managerial and economic factors that can make eHealth a successful and sustainable venture for healthcare organisations and governments. Consumer and patient involvement at the stage of decision-making and planning may enhance implementation of patient-centred applications.

It is possible that eHealth sustainability requires synergic action between the private and public sector. Such partnership models may enhance planning beyond the technology level and facilitate systems and problem-solving for the sustainable and integrated use of eHealth.

A comprehensive model of this kind, originally proposed by Beauchamp [42] as a generic business plan, was adapted by Catwell and Sheikh [20] for the purposes of examining how eHealth could be made more sustainable, focusing on the problems of patients, families and clinicians rather than on the technical problems alone. Conditions in most countries are not yet mature enough to enable healthcare systems to undertake such implementation. The model proposes a way to facilitate change management and sustainable use for future eHealth initiatives. The central element of the plan is the statement of a problem (e.g. why is change from paper-based to electronic medical records needed?) that needs a solution and subsequent facilitation steps that form a 'chain of reasoning' that lead to how eHealth can provide the solution [20].

In Table 18.2, we have mapped out the seven steps with the example of shifting from paper-based records to records available to all parties electronically. This example illustrates the potential of eHealth to benefit patients, clinicians and health services, but also the risks associated with

Table 18.2 Seven-step sustainability plan.

Steps	Statement of the problem	Purpose/objective
1. Drivers (definition of problem)	Why is change needed?	Develop records that allow multiple-user, efficient and secure access to patient records when needed
2. Vision	What would be the possible responses to those drivers; i.e. what will the revised model of delivering care look like?	Patient records will be readily accessible from anywhere within the healthcare institution/setting
3. Goals	How will a project move towards realising this vision?	Electronic health records will be deployed through a web-based secure network
4. Business objectives	How will success be measured?	Healthcare professionals, patients, their caregivers and the public at large will have access to efficient electronic health information over a secure network, from anywhere at any time, within *x* years at *y* cost. It is important that these timelines and costs are realistic
5. Business require-ments	What capabilities will be needed in order to achieve these business objectives?	Detailed technical specifications, access to authority, social (i.e. behavioural and organisational) changes
6. Design	What are the possible solutions to meet the need and the requirements identified in the previous step?	Commissioning of a custom-made web-based electronic health record system
7. Solution	Have the problems been resolved and the anticipated benefits realised within the proposed timescale and allocated budget?	Propose a plan for continuous evaluation

Source: Adapted from [20]. (With permission.)

privacy and confidentiality and the challenge of installing new systems that cross institutional borders.

The above model should consider needs at practice level and be adjusted so as to facilitate not only effective implementation of sustainable eHealth solutions, such as electronic health records, but also the realisation of targeted health outcomes (such as diabetes management in an endocrinology clinic and cholesterol management in a cardiology clinic). A targeted health outcome is integral in defining the problem, purpose and objective at all stages of the seven-step sustainability plan.

Finally, long-term sustainability of eHealth will materialise only if applications provide substantial maximisation of benefits and minimisation of clinical risk to patients. There is no reason why eHealth should not be subjected to the same rigorous evaluation of effectiveness and safety as other clinical and pharmacologic interventions. Nevertheless, the creation of a solid evidence base that is intervention specific is a major challenge, and requires the investment of time, effort and resources.

References

1. Gupta A (2008 October 20) Prescription for change: health care has managed to avoid the information-technology revolution. But it won't for much longer. *The Wall Street Journal*, R6.
2. Dansky KH, Thompson D, Sanner T (2006) A framework for evaluating eHealth research. *Evaluation and Program Planning* **29**, 397–404.
3. Eysenbach G (2001) What is e-health? *Journal of Medical Internet Research* **3**, e20.
4. Pagliari C, Sloan D, Gregor P, et al. (2005) What is eHealth (4): a scoping exercise to map the field. *Journal of Medical Internet Research* **7**, e9.
5. Maheu M, Whitten P, Allen A (2001) *E-Health, Telehealth, and Telemedicine*. Jossey Bass, San Francisco.
6. Oh H, Rizo C, Enkin M, Jadad A (2005) What is eHealth (3): a systematic review of published definitions. *Journal of Medical Internet Research* **7**, e1.
7. Wilson P, Leitner C, Moussalli A (2004) Mapping the potential of eHealth: empowering the citizen through eHealth tools and services. *eHealth Conference*, 5–6 May 2004, Cork, Ireland.
8. Blobel B, Kalra D, Koehn M, et al. (2009) The role of ontologies for sustainable, semantically interoperable and trustworthy EHR solutions. *Studies in Health Technology and Informatics* **150**, 953–957.
9. Bickford C, Hunter K (2006) Theories, models, and frameworks. In: Saba V, McCormick K, (eds.) *Essentials of Nursing Informatics*. McGraw-Hill, New York.
10. Shekelle P, Morton S, Keeler E (2006) *Costs and Benefits of Health Information Technology*. Agency for Healthcare Research and Quality, Rockville.
11. Mekhjian HS, Kumar RR, Kuehn L, et al. (2002) Immediate benefits realized following implementation of physician order entry at an academic medical center. *Journal of the American Medical Informatics Association* **9**, 529–539.
12. Kreuter MW, Caburnay CA, Chen JJ, Donlin MJ (2004) Effectiveness of individually tailored calendars in promoting childhood immunization in urban public health centers. *American Journal of Public Health and the Nation's Health* **94**, 122–127.
13. Marcus AM, Wolfe M, Rimer P, et al. (2003) Understanding the normalization of telemedicine services through qualitative evaluation. *Journal of the American Medical Informatics Association* **10**, 596–604.
14. Smeets T, Brug J, de Vries H (2008) Effects of tailoring health messages on physical activity. *Health Education Research* **23**, 402–413.
15. Pagliari C, Detmer D, Singleton P (2007) *Electronic Personal Health Records Emergence and Implications for the UK*. Available from: http://www.nuffieldtrust.org.uk/ecomm/files/Elec%20Personal%20Records%20II.pdf. Accessed: 18 February 2010.
16. Car J, Sheikh A (2004) Email consultations in health care: 1 – scope and effectiveness. *British Medical Journal* **329**, 435–438.

17. Car J, Ng C, Atun R, Card A (2008) SMS text message healthcare appointment reminders in England. *The Journal of Ambulatory Care Management* **31**, 216–219.
18. Car J, Koshy E, Bell D, Sheikh A (2008) Telephone triage in out of hours call centres. *British Medical Journal* **337**, a1167.
19. Lustria ML, Cortese J, Noar SM, Glueckauf RL (2009) Computer-tailored health interventions delivered over the Web: review and analysis of key components. *Patient Education and Counseling* **74**, 156–173.
20. Catwell L, Sheikh A (2009) Evaluating eHealth interventions: the need for continuous systemic evaluation. *Public Library of Science Medicine* **6**, e1000126.
21. World Bank (1996) *The World Bank Participation Sourcebook.* Available from: http://www-wds.worldbank.org/external/default/WDSContentServer/WDSP/IB/1996/02/01/000009265_3961214175537/Rendered/PDF/multi_page.pdf. Accessed: 17 August 2009.
22. Commission of the European Communities (2004) *e-Health – Making Healthcare Better for European Citizens: An Action Plan for a European e-Health Area.* Available from: http://eur-lex.europa.eu/LexUriServ/LexUriServ.do?uri=COM:2004:0356:FIN:EN:PDF. Accessed: 22 July 2009.
23. Ammenwerth E, Shaw NT (2005) Bad health informatics can kill – is evaluation the answer? *Methods of Information in Medicine* **44**, 1–3.
24. Chiauzzi E, Green TC, Lord S, Thum C, Goldstein M (2005) My student body: a high-risk drinking prevention web site for college students. *Journal of American College Health* **53**, 263–274.
25. Oenema A, Brug J, Lechner L (2001) Web-based tailored nutrition education: results of a randomized controlled trial. *Health Education Research* **16**, 647–660.
26. Strecher VJ, Shiffman S, West R (2005) Randomized controlled trial of a web-based computer-tailored smoking cessation program as a supplement to nicotine patch therapy. *Addiction* **100**, 682–688.
27. Jimison H, Gorman P, Woods S, et al. (2008) *Barriers and Drivers of Health Information Technology Use for the Elderly, Chronically Ill, and Underserved. Evidence Report/Technology Assessment.* Agency for Healthcare Research and Quality, Rockville.
28. Mudur G (2004) The great technological divide. *British Medical Journal* **328**, 788.
29. Han YY, Carcillo JA, Venkataraman ST, et al. (2005) Unexpected increased mortality after implementation of a commercially sold computerized physician order entry system. *Pediatrics* **116**, 1506–1512.
30. Pappas Y, Seale C (2010) The physical examination in telecardiology and televascular consultations: a study using conversation analysis. *Patient Education and Counseling* **81**, 113–118.
31. Alastair B (2009) *eHealth Pathway Analysis: eHealth Enabled Process Improvement.* eHealth Change and Benefits Division, Edinburgh. Available from: http://www.ehealth.scot.nhs.uk/secure/Pathway%20Analysis%20Tool%20v1%202.pdf. Accessed: 21 November 2009.
32. Pappas Y, Seale C (2009) The opening phase of telemedicine consultations: an analysis of interaction. *Social Science & Medicine* **68**, 1229–1237.
33. Parker J, Coiera E (2000) Improving clinical communication: a view from psychology. *Journal of the American Medical Informatics Association* **7**, 453–461.
34. Goldstein MK, Hoffman BB, Coleman RW, et al. (2001) Patient safety in guideline-based decision support for hypertension management: ATHENA DSS. *Journal of the American Medical Informatics Association* **9**, S11–S16, 214–218.

35. Stead W, Lin H (eds) (2009) *Computational Technology for Effective Health Care: Immediate Steps and Strategic Directions*. National Academics Press, Washington DC. Sciences
36. Rodrigues R (2008) Compelling issues for adoption of e-health. *The Commonwealth Health Ministers Reference Book 2008*. Available from: http://www.ehealthstrategies.com/files/Commonwealth_MOH_Apr08.pdf. Accessed: 23 March 2011
37. Ammenwerth E, Brender J, Nykanen P, Prokosch HU, Rigby M, Talmon J (2004) Visions and strategies to improve evaluation of health information systems. Reflections and lessons based on the HIS-EVAL workshop in Innsbruck. *International Journal of Medical Informatics* **73**, 479–491.
38. Atherton H, Car J, Meyer B (2009) Email for the provision of information on disease prevention and health promotion (Protocol). *Cochrane Database of Systematic Reviews*, CD007982.
39. Colledge A, Car J, Majeed A (2008) Interventions for enhancing the skills of consumers to find, evaluate and use online health information (Protocol). *Cochrane Database of Systematic Reviews*, CD007092.
40. May C, Harrison R, MacFarlane A, Williams T, Mair F, Wallace P (2003) Why do telemedicine systems fail to normalize as stable models of service delivery? *Journal of Telemedicine and Telecare* **9**(Suppl. 1), S25–S26.
41. Finch T, May C, Mair F, Mort M, Gask L (2003) Integrating service development with evaluation in telehealthcare: an ethnographic study. *British Medical Journal* **327**, 1205–1209.
42. Beauchamp G (2007) *Business Analysis – Delivering the Right Solution to the Right Problem*. Available from: http://www.businessanalystsolutions.com/BA%20Chain%20of%20Reasoning.pdf. Accessed: 22 August 2009.

Index

Note: Page numbers with italicized *b*'s, *f*'s and *t*'s refer to boxes, figures, and tables

The Knowledgeable Patient: Communication and Participation in Health – A Cochrane Handbook, First Edition. Edited by Sophie Hill.